W21
26/3/14

ROYAL SOCIETY of MEDICINE Career Handbook

FY1 | ST2

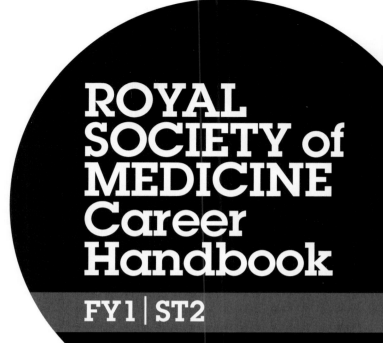

ROYAL SOCIETY of MEDICINE Career Handbook

FY1 | ST2

By **Muhunthan Thillai** and **Kaji Sritharan**

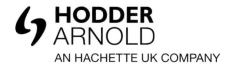

HODDER ARNOLD
AN HACHETTE UK COMPANY

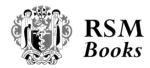

RSM Books

First published in Great Britain in 2011 by
Hodder Arnold, an imprint of Hodder Education, a division of Hachette UK,
338 Euston Road, London NW1 3BH

http://www.hodderarnold.com

Hachette UK's policy is to use papers that are natural, renewable and recyclable products
and made from wood grown in sustainable forests. The logging and manufacturing
processes are expected to conform to the environmental regulations of the country of origin.

Whilst the advice and information in this book are believed to be true and accurate at the date
of going to press, neither the author[s] nor the publisher can accept any legal responsibility
or liability for any errors or omissions that may be made. In particular, (but without limiting
the generality of the preceding disclaimer) every effort has been made to check drug dosages;
however it is still possible that errors have been missed. Furthermore, dosage schedules are
constantly being revised and new side-effects recognized. For these reasons the reader is
strongly urged to consult the drug companies' printed instructions before administering any
of the drugs recommended in this book.

British Library Cataloguing in Publication Data
A catalogue record for this book is available from the British Library

Library of Congress Cataloging-in-Publication Data
A catalog record for this book is available from the Library of Congress

ISBN   978-1-853-15927-5

1 2 3 4 5 6 7 8 9 10

Publisher: Caroline Makepeace
Editorial Manager: Francesca Naish
Production Controller: Kate Harris
Cover Design: Helen Townson
Project managed by Naughton Project Management

Cover image © Tim Vernon, LTH NHS Trust/Science Photo Library

The logo of the Royal Society of Medicine is a registered trade mark, which it has licensed to
Hodder Arnold.
Typeset in 10/14 pt Serifa-Roman by MPS Limited, a Macmillan Company
Printed and bound in the UK by CPI Antony Rowe Ltd

What do you think about this book? Or any other Hodder Arnold title?
Please visit our website: www.hodderarnold.com

For my parents. My father, who taught me mathematics on our Dining room table in Westaway Court, and my mother, who passed onto me her love of books.

Muhunthan Thillai
Jersey

Acknowledgements

We are extremely grateful to Dr Andrew Papanikitas for his contribution to Chapter 3: Getting through the Foundation Years and Chapter 5: Specialty Training Application forms, as well as his authorship of Chapter 7: GP Recruitment.

Foreword

During my own time at medical school I went to a conference in Switzerland. I made friends with a bunch of Norwegian medics who suggested that we climbed a nearby mountain together, which sounded like a terrific idea. I had no idea what I was letting myself in for. I soon leaned that Norwegians run up mountains like lesser mortals pop out to get some milk. Well, I suppose they had more mountains to practice on than I had. However I made it, and I think I managed to pretend not to be completely exhausted by trying to keep up. And the view from the top was worth it. I would have done a jolly sight better had I understood from the outset what was involved, and if I had been better prepared.

A career in medicine takes longer than climbing a mountain. Otherwise the same principles apply. Determination and hard work are taken for granted. But preparation will score much better than blundering along. Understanding the map of the terrain and how best to jump the hurdles really is a good idea. The good news is that the view is immensely worthwhile at all parts of the journey, and you will make some terrific friends along the way. Medicine is a demanding career, but most of those who go for it would not be satisfied with less.

Hippocrates wrote that the 'art [of medicine] is long but life is short'. I suspect he wrote that when he was old. When you start out a professional lifetime probably seems long, and the journey within medicine to the summit of a career may seem lost in the clouds. But the frantic pace of a medical career will see the years passing by quickly enough. We only have one shot at life, and one shot at a medical career – it's not a dress rehearsal. Medicine is a mountain range with so many possibilities, so many different peaks and viewpoints. Thillai and Sritharan have drawn up a superb set of maps for the medical climber. There is not one right way to do it, but for any one medic there will be better ways and also less successful ways. This book should be a terrific help to ensure that you make the most of your one shot at this fantastic career.

Some of the individual pathways in medicine seem very different now from a decade ago, never mind when I qualified at the end of the 1970s. MMC has represented a big shift in the training culture. It is far from a perfect system, however it has settled down a lot from its turbulent early days, and is certainly stable enough to believe that now is a good time to be drawing up the sort of maps that Thillai and Sritharan have given us here. We may well see changes in the F1 and F2 years following Professor John Collins' excellent and thought provoking report into the Foundation years[1]. But there will always be changes, for in medicine change is here to stay. However there are also some constant principles that will determine your success. Hard work, applied intelligence and moral courage always show through in the end. There is no easy drive up these mountains.

If there is one other thing you should attend to at every point of your own climb that is the voice of the patient. Medicine offers this wide mountain range of different possibilities. As an intellectual discipline it encompasses both high end science and the humanities. As an activity it spans the highly academic and the very practical. One thing should hold the whole thing together and that is our concern for patients. Medics form a wide and diverse community, a community with space for many different personalities and skills, but with a shared aim. Unless we do this climbing for the good of our patients then we do it with no morally valid aim. If we put the interest of the patient at the centre not just because the GMC say we should, but because we ourselves *must*, then the view really is terrific. We will go through difficult times, and of course we will witness some difficult, even terrible, events happening to our patients. If we know we are doing this for a worthwhile purpose, a purpose that has a thread of moral value running through it even when we are too tired to remember this, then we have every reason to believe that we really are a part of the greatest profession in the world.

I hope you are able to use this book to make the most of the opportunities before you. And I wish you every success, both professionally and personally, in the years ahead.

David Misselbrook
Dean
Royal Society of Medicine

---

1 Collins J. Foundation for Excellence. An evaluation of the Foundation Programme. Medical Education England, October 2010.

Contents

Introduction

Graduate students starting their MBA at Harvard Business School are told from the outset that getting the prestigious qualification is just the start. It is not a final destination but merely a transition that prepares them for the rest of their career. Along with lectures on corporate finance, global markets and emerging economies, there is a specific module dedicated to developing a vision for their own future and devoting all their energy towards achieving that goal.

Medical students have an equally intensive undergraduate study. They are taught human anatomy, molecular biology and statistics. They spend time on the wards learning how to deal with a number of different systemic diseases but somewhere along the way they miss out on the teaching that is fundamental to a student of business.

How should a final-year student choose what career to pursue and what do they need to do to get into that career? What sort of questions are asked on an application form, and what type of answers are the shortlisting panel looking for? How should you prepare yourself for an interview? If you are offered a place that would not be your first choice should you accept it immediately and then work towards the greater goal or should you risk being without a job in the short term rather than doing something that takes you away from your ideal career?

Attaining your own career goals in medicine in the UK was, until relatively recently, very much a lottery. Jobs were advertised in a few select journals and candidates could apply for as many or as few as they wanted. They could be announced at any time of year and deaneries across the country placed advertisements at different times. It was easy to miss a dream job simply because you hadn't read the current issue of *BMJ Careers*.

Candidates were chosen for interview based on a curriculum vitae, which could range from one side of paper to a ream of pages stapled at the top and placed in a binder. Those who used yellow parchment paper may have stood out from those who printed theirs off on plain white paper.

Shortlisting for a job interview was sometimes about who you knew, rather than how much you knew. Career advancement in many fields often meant socialising with your boss and colleagues outside of working hours. In some respects things have perhaps changed very little but in others there have been dramatic differences over time.

It was unlikely that candidates for junior training jobs had any research experience or had carried out an audit. It was even less likely that they could answer a question about *fitness to practice* or the current changes within the National Health Service. An interview question about their experience as a vascular surgeon may have been answered well but a query about the seven pillars of clinical governance might have been met with a blank look.

The advent of Modernising Medical Careers has changed all of this. Jobs are now advertised at specific time points throughout the year and almost all applications are made online. It is not good enough to have merely helped with an audit or written a poster. The candidates who are selected for interview will have initiated an audit and then claimed that it had far-reaching conclusions. Rather than being an author on a poster they may have helped produce it and then presented the results to a regional specialist meeting.

The world of min-CEX, DOPs and 360-degree appraisals may have improved the process of review and competency but it does have a number of downsides. Perhaps chief amongst these is the difficulty of standing out from the crowd. If all applicants have an up-to-date training portfolio then how do you show a shortlisting committee that you are better than your peers? If all candidates have participated in an audit then how do you convince the interview panel that yours was one of the better ones?

The answer is to follow the example of the MBA student. You need to have a long-term strategy and then devote your resources towards achieving that aim. The effort that you put in towards your career goals at the outset will have far-reaching benefits and short-term pain does indeed often lead to advantages in the long term. No matter whether you wish to be a part-time salaried GP in a remote village in the Cotswolds or an academic neurosurgeon in a London teaching hospital, it still pays to have a strategy.

You need to understand the exact questions on an application form and know what the panel is looking for to achieve maximum marks. You need to practice your interview answers until you know what to say even before they have finished asking you the question. When offered to initiate an audit or a piece of research by a senior colleague you need to know when to accept and devote an entire weekend to making a deadline and when to simply say no and walk away.

Many of these questions can only be answered with experience. You need to spend time working as a doctor and speak to senior colleagues who have faced these challenges before. You will get conflicting advice about how to pursue your career and at the end of the day it is important that you make your own decisions based on what you understand and what is important to you. We hope, however, that this book will help point you in the right direction.

In the words of Harvard's MBA programme, "It's time to find your future".

Muhunthan Thillai & Kaji Sritharan
London

1

How to choose your specialty

Key aims of this chapter

- Outline general considerations for all careers
- Discuss how to prioritise a career with the rest of your life
- Detail advantages and disadvantages of specific career paths.

Introduction

The majority of students starting medical school will have little idea as to what field they will eventually pursue. Even for those who do, the choice often changes over time. A student ambitious enough to want a career as an internationally renowned heart surgeon may end their foundation years dreaming of becoming a GP in a small village and vice versa. However, as most students progress through medical school they start to have some idea of the type of career and lifestyle that is available to them.

Medical careers can be vastly different to each other in a huge number of aspects including time spent at work, time in training, need for research, postgraduate qualifications and on-call commitments. Even the pay can be astoundingly different. A cardiologist practising in a city teaching hospital with a large private practice may end up earning ten times as much as a colleague from medical school who is a salaried GP in the same region.

All of these factors need to be considered before embarking on your chosen career. However, not all aspects of your career can be planned out in advance. Serendipity plays a large part and doctors can end up specialising in a field for the most unusual reasons, e.g. meeting an inspiring consultant at a conference or the need to move closer to one set of grandparents after starting a family. Whatever the reasons, it is vital to have an idea of what is involved before coming to a decision that will affect the rest of your life.

General considerations with all careers

Job satisfaction

At the heart of choosing your career is the concept of job satisfaction. This can be affected by a number of things from how busy an 'on call' is to how much income there is to be gained from private practice. When these factors are combined the ideal job should still leave you with a sense of satisfaction. The only real way to gauge this is to try to experience the field for yourself. Medical school attachments will give some idea but it is often not until you work in a field as a junior doctor that you truly realise what it is like.

It can be relatively straightforward to exclude some careers, e.g. someone who does not like working with their hands would not choose surgery and a person who wants to work within a multidisciplinary setting may not be suited to life as a microbiologist. Making your choice of final career can be difficult and it is important to speak to as many people as possible before making this decision. Try and find out as many disadvantages of the career as you can and make sure that you can live with them before deciding if it is the correct career for you.

Workload

Although it is generally accepted that doctors work pretty hard, within the profession, there is a wide range of the exact amount of work carried out. Doctors that are at the same stage in their career and earning the same pay may work completely different amounts of time. For junior doctors, this in theory has been standardised with the European Working Time Directive but in reality the actual hours worked by both trainees and consultants can vary dramatically.

As well as the hours worked, the intensity of the work needs to be taken into account. Specialist trainees in emergency medicine may find themselves on their feet all day seeing patients continuously with limited time for breaks. An equivalent trainee in respiratory medicine may actually find that when providing ward cover they can conduct a ward round at a more leisurely pace, assign the jobs to their more junior team members and spend some time reading or catching up on paperwork.

The type of institution can also dramatically change the workload. For example, a general medicine trainee in a large teaching hospital will typically be on call with a number of junior colleagues and may end up reviewing and admitting only a small number of patients within an on-call period. The same trainee in a district general hospital may find that they have to see far more patients when on-call due to both the reduced level of support and the increased numbers of potential patients within their catchment area. The same differences may apply at a consultant level.

On-call commitments are also very different. An ophthalmology trainee will do an on-call shift from home and may be able to deal with most calls they receive over the telephone. A general surgery trainee at the same hospital may have to be resident on-call and physically be present to review sick patients and make decisions about taking them to theatre. The commitments may be different between trainee and consultant and so it is worth noting that a demanding period of specialist training may pay off with less arduous on-call commitments as a consultant or other senior doctor.

Things are, however, changing and it is vital to find out about long-term plans within a specialty. Consultants who may have traditionally been at home may find themselves staying in hospitals, e.g. interventional cardiologists may have to commit to a resident on-call rota to deal with primary angioplasties in the middle of the night.

Income

Whilst doctors are supposed to be completely altruistic, the rewards for hard work are usually happily accepted. Such pay can vary dramatically and must be taken into account. If planning for a lavish lifestyle with large houses, fast cars and tropical holidays then your chosen career may not pay the way. However, those with more modest expectations find that most careers will pay enough.

A choice faced by most junior doctors is whether to go into primary or secondary care. Hospital doctors who make it to the position of consultant are often paid well but partners in a general practice can earn even more than hospital consultants, sometimes with a smaller workload. More junior salaried GPs can also be better paid than specialist trainees but the potential for increased earnings above the standard salary by specialist doctors is often greater than with GPs.

Hospital specialists and GPs can supplement their salary in a number of ways. Pay awards and discretionary points for specialists in the

National Health Service (NHS) can almost double a standard salary. These awards are given in stages and can be made at a local or national level. There are guidelines as to who can apply and when they can apply and the criteria for such pay increases include commitments to research, teaching and management.

Specialists can opt for private practice to supplement their income. Hospital consultants will have fixed times during the week when they are allowed to see private patients, either in the outpatient setting, or as inpatients on a private ward or in a private hospital. The potential for private income is limited in some fields whereas those in areas with interventional work can be hugely rewarded for their work and it is important to take this into consideration. Some doctors may elect to see private patients after standard working hours but this can obviously have a negative impact on other aspects of their life.

Aside from seeing private patients, there are numerous other ways to supplement an income but these will vary between specialties. For example, a medical doctor who practices as a part-time GP may be able to earn a second salary as a medical journalist. A general medical staff grade doctor may be able to act as an advisor to medical insurance companies and an academic consultant could sit on the board of a pharmaceutical company. Alternative positions such as these may have ethical implications and may also take up a large amount of time, all of which have to be considered.

Education and learning

All careers within medicine require life-long learning but again the amount involved is highly variable. A specialist within a surgical field may find that he has to keep up-to-date with the latest procedures by attending conferences, practical teaching sessions with industry and hands-on learning with more experienced specialists. This type of continual learning may not be suited to all and a clinician may prefer a specialty where the evidence for practice is less subject to change and hence there is less to keep up with.

In addition, careers in some fields will allow for teaching medical students and junior doctors, e.g. a gastroenterology consultant in a teaching hospital may have several junior doctors and a continuous stream of medical students whereas a palliative care consultant in the same teaching hospital may have only one junior doctor and the occasional student on a specialist placement. The concept of passing on knowledge to juniors may strongly appeal to some but may be regarded by others as too time consuming and not for them.

There has been a deliberate attempt not to discuss Modernising Medical Careers (MMC) within this chapter. This is because the process is still evolving. Although it does not have a direct bearing on specialist careers in terms of endpoints, it does have an impact on training in terms of job competition and workforce planning, nationalising of training schemes and workload. These must be taken into account when choosing a specialty, e.g. if a particular specialty training programme is advertised at a national level and there is a high number of applicants to positions then this must be considered.

Completion of specialist training does not guarantee a consultant post in all hospital specialties. There is a surplus of trainees at the end of their training in some specialties and the demand for posts may necessitate research degrees, Fellowships or further experience at a junior level before appointment. For current and up-to-date information regarding MMC, follow the links found at the MMC website (www.mmc.nhs.uk).

Box 1.1 A note about Modernising Medical Careers and job competition

Prioritising a career with the rest of your life

Part-time medicine

There is an increasing ability to both train and specialise part time or flexibly in most medical fields. Once a domain almost exclusively for women there is now a significant number of men who wish to practice part time but when applying for such training the deanery will need a strong reason. This may be that you wish to start a family or look after young children or it may be because you wish to pursue a second but related career, e.g. a junior doctor in psychiatry who wishes to use his experience in medical journalism to write for a medical magazine may be allowed to train in this way. Some doctors may want to train part time from the moment they enter specialist training whereas others may wish to complete a more demanding period of training before starting as a specialist part time.

The obvious advantage of a part-time career is that it enables you to pursue something else in addition to medicine. There are some downsides that need to be considered before making this decision. A part-time job means a part-time salary that may in reality be less than half of what is earned by colleagues. In addition, there needs to be strong continuity of care, e.g. two consultants job sharing and dealing with medical inpatients need to communicate well to hand over the care in the middle of the week. Doctors who job share must have a similar work ethos as differences in commitment to the department and to patients can have a hugely damaging effect on working relationships.

Travel

Doctors in training may be in a relationship or at the stage of having or starting a family. The amount of travel involved with posts must therefore be taken into account. Some deaneries in the UK are far larger than others and specialist trainee posts may be too far apart to commute from home. This is made more difficult in certain specialties such as neurosurgery, where centres for training may be extremely far away from each other. The combination of two careers with children starting school may mean that rather than moving an entire family across the region you will have to live apart for periods of time.

This is not a viable option for everyone and it may be possible for two doctors in a relationship to link their applications so that they work in the same region, at the same time, if they are at the same point in their career. Inter-deanery transfers are also possible but transfer into the more popular regions is competitive and may require an application to a formal board. Some careers may require academic qualifications or travel for Fellowships abroad before getting enough experience to apply for a specialist position and this also needs to be taken into account.

Teaching centre or district general hospital

Hospital doctors working in teaching hospitals and GPs associated with universities may find that their work–life balance is very different from that of their colleagues elsewhere. For example, a medical consultant in a teaching hospital may have a smaller caseload in terms of inpatient and outpatient clinics than her counterpart in a smaller district general hospital. However, the other responsibilities associated with a teaching hospital position may mean a greater commitment to her work in terms of hours spent in the hospital as well as work taken home.

These commitments may include research proposals for funding, reviewing experimental results from an academic collaboration, teaching medical students both by the bedside and in lectures, and management issues associated with being attached to a university. Whilst such responsibilities may result in a higher pay, the time commitment needed can be heavy and must be taken into account when choosing where to practice medicine.

Private practice

Seeing patients privately can be financially rewarding but does have negative aspects. The major problem is to do with time. As well as seeing patients during typical office hours it may be necessary to hold evening clinics or operate at the weekend in order to meet your financial expectations.

The increased workload involved is not confined solely to time spent with patients. It may be that as a specialist looking after an inpatient there are no juniors that can help and only a skeleton staff on-call at night and at the weekends. If patients become unwell during these times, then you may be expected to return to deal with them prior to their transfer to a more acute medical setting.

Dealing with insurance companies and litigation can also be demanding and this needs to be taken into account when deciding on a specialty. It may be that you choose not to practice private medicine at all no matter what specialty you work in, but the pressure to do so in terms of potential financial rewards can be too great to resist.

Non-consultant posts and salaried GPs

The commitments needed to practice as a hospital consultant or GP partner may be too great for some in terms of juggling interests or commitments outside medicine. A consultant may have to take paperwork from his management responsibilities home to finish at the weekend, which could stop him spending quality time with his children, or a GP partner may find that she is spending long hours on site after seeing patients simply to finish the paperwork associated with running a practice.

One way around this is to practice in alternative posts. An associate specialist in hospital medicine may receive a similar basic salary to that of a hospital consultant but be able to practice without the same managerial and administrative responsibilities associated with a consultant position. Alternatively, a salaried GP may earn less than that of a partner in the same practice but have far fewer non-clinical responsibilities.

Thoughts about specific career paths

The information in this section is by no means exhaustive. Although it covers the majority of UK specialties it does not cover them all. In addition, advantages of some jobs may be seen as disadvantages by others, e.g. a clinician may find it advantageous not to have to do resident on-calls whereas his colleague may find that they would rather be on-call and enjoy seeing acutely unwell patients. Some doctors may relish the opportunity to have lengthy multidisciplinary team meetings whereas others may find them time consuming.

A number of advantages and disadvantages have been suggested for each of the major specialties. They are taken from postgraduate college information, reviews of the specialty and discussions with specialists in these fields. There are, of course, certain caveats to the information, e.g. 'office hours' do not mean a straightforward 9-to-5 job but instead indicate that compared to some other specialties, the trainees and senior doctors get to start work and leave to go home at a more reasonable time.

The approach taken to summarising the pros and cons of a career are to assume that you are a typical foundation year 1 (FY1 or F1) doctor who has just graduated, i.e. you are keen to learn, want a varied and stimulating life with a decent salary yet have a good work–life balance.

Of course, nobody is typical.

Table 1.1: Pros and cons of different specialties

Specialty	Pros	Cons
Anaesthetics	<ul><li>Fast-paced and intensive lifestyle</li><li>Large array of general medicine, surgery and paediatrics to deal with on a daily basis</li><li>Flexible training programmes with job sharing at a senior level</li></ul>	<ul><li>Consultants frequently have to work nights and weekends to deal with critical cases</li><li>Trainees work a large number of shifts and are often asked to help other teams to look after ill patients, which can be demanding</li><li>Less continuity of care than for other specialties</li></ul>
Cardiology	<ul><li>An invasive specialty with a large number of procedures with potentially immediate clinical results</li><li>Opportunity for large private practice</li><li>Dedicated research funding with ongoing opportunities for academic work and teaching</li></ul>	<ul><li>Competition for both training and consultant posts is currently higher than in other medical specialties</li><li>Advent of primary angioplasty centres means interventional consultants may have to be resident on-call</li><li>Combined workload of NHS and private patients can be demanding</li></ul>

Specialty	Pros	Cons
Cardiothoracic surgery	<ul><li>An invasive specialty with a large number of procedures with potentially immediate clinical results</li><li>Opportunity for private practice with caveat of decreasing demand</li><li>Ability to tell people that you are a 'heart surgeon'</li></ul>	<ul><li>Competition for both training and consultant posts is currently higher than in other surgical specialties</li><li>Increasing amount of interventional work by cardiologists and radiologists means a decrease in demand for surgical services</li><li>Combined workload of NHS and private operations can be demanding</li></ul>
Care of the elderly	<ul><li>Consultant posts are slightly less competitive than with other medical specialties</li><li>Wide variety of general medicine encountered on a daily basis</li><li>Potential for increased academic research with an ageing population</li></ul>	<ul><li>Less potential for private practice than in some other medical specialties</li><li>Potentially heavy workload</li><li>Strong multidisciplinary approach to care may not suit all clinicians</li></ul>
Dermatology	<ul><li>Good potential for private practice</li><li>Increasing number of practical procedures</li><li>An office-based specialty with minimal chance of having to go in on-call either as a trainee or a consultant</li></ul>	<ul><li>Less funding for academic work than some other specialties</li><li>Competition for both training and consultant posts is currently higher than in other medical specialties</li><li>Largely outpatient based with fewer emergencies than other medical specialties</li></ul>
Emergency medicine & Acute medicine	<ul><li>Varied working day with potential for stimulating and difficult cases</li><li>Current expansion of the specialty means an increasing number of training positions</li><li>As a relatively new specialty there is ample space for clinical research</li><li>Consultants are currently off site when on-call and are less likely to have to come in than those in other specialties</li></ul>	<ul><li>Large amount of shift work as a middle-grade doctor</li><li>Work can be physically and emotionally draining</li><li>Limited opportunity for private practice</li><li>Lack of continuity of care with specialist teams often receiving the thanks of a patient and their family</li></ul>

(Continued)

Table 1.1: Continued.

Specialty	Pros	Cons
Endocrinology	• Complex spectrum of medicine is encountered in everyday practice • Good scope for academic research • Potential for financially lucrative links with industry in chronic diseases of high prevalence, e.g. diabetes	• Hugely multidisciplinary specialty that may not suit all • Largely outpatient based with fewer emergencies than other medical specialties • Large number of academics in post, meaning that research is often needed to secure consultant posts
ENT surgery	• Wide spectrum of acute and chronic conditions to be treated • Large caseload of paediatric patients may appeal to some surgeons • Good potential for private practice	• Large number of outpatient appointments and procedures compared to some other surgical specialties, which may not be suited to all • More emphasis currently on further specialist training than some of the other surgical specialties • Long and complex operations and operating times are not suited to all
Gastroenterology	• Large potential for interventional work, which is replacing surgery in many cases • Private work is more lucrative than in most other medical specialties • Increasing tendency towards high-tech medicine, e.g. capsule endoscopies	• Consultants will increasingly have to come in on call to deal with emergency patients who require interventional work • Like in some other medical specialties it has a significant amount of chronic patients with difficult-to-diagnose diseases • Potential for loss of skills as endoscopies are taken over by specialist nurses and GPs
General practice	• Opportunity for prolonged continuity of care • Partners start on salaries equivalent to (or higher than) hospital consultants • Ability to opt out of evening and weekend duties • Flexible training programmes with job sharing at a senior level • Training available for those who wish to offer a specialist service	• Increasing difficulties in getting partnerships means many GPs are opting for a fixed salary, which is often lower than that of a partner • Administrative paperwork is regarded as more substantial than that for hospital doctors • Less opportunity for collaborative academic work than in hospital medicine

Specialty	Pros	Cons
General surgery	• Varied working day with potential for stimulating and difficult cases • Good scope for private practice • Ability to fix a problem with relatively instant success • Increasing use of high-tech surgery to perform routine operations e.g. specialised endoscopic surgery	• Consultants may be called in to work nights and weekends to deal with critical cases • May have to work long hours to operate on ill patients • Training programmes can be challenging, particularly with the reduction in hours due to the European Working Time Directive
Genitourinary and HIV medicine	• Wide spectrum of general medicine is encountered • Office hours with low chance of having to come in when on call as a consultant • Strong potential for academic work	• Potential for busy caseload in outpatient clinics • Limited opportunity for private practice • Increasing administrative workload
Haematology	• Office hours with low chance of having to come in when on-call as a consultant • Strong history of academic work • Rapid potential for new technologies and treatments to cure otherwise fatal conditions	• Competition for both training and consultant posts is currently high with academic work often required • Postgraduate exams are generally accepted as being harder than some other specialties • Critically ill young patients who were previously well can be challenging both medically and emotionally
Infectious diseases	• Potential for overseas travel as part of training programme • Huge variety of general medical knowledge needed to make it a varied and interesting specialty • May be no acute medical on-call commitments as a consultant	• Large number of academics in post, meaning that research is often necessary to secure consultant posts • Limited opportunity for private practice • Limited number of consultant posts in the UK mean some doctors end up combining it with other fields, e.g. acute medicine

(Continued)

How to Choose Your Specialty | 11

Specialty	Pros	Cons
Intensive care medicine	• Varied training with entry into field from medicine or anaesthesia • Very acute work initially with doctors dealing with critically ill patients • Encompasses a large amount of medicine and surgery as part of the training and practice	• Long hours and resident on-calls as trainees • Consultants may have to come in to see critically ill patients (from other teams) to a greater degree than in other specialties • Limited potential for private practice
Medical oncology and Clinical oncology	• Strong potential for academic work with dedicated funding streams • Consultants and most trainees are currently often off-site when on-call and are less likely to have to come in than in other specialties • Increasing technologies and scientific knowledge are constantly pushing the boundaries of patient care	• Postgraduate exams are generally accepted as being harder than in some other specialties with some knowledge of maths and physics required • Working with cancer patients can be emotionally draining • Competition for both training and consultant posts is currently high with academic research often required
Microbiology Immunology Biochemistry Pathology	• Varied working day with interaction with a number of clinical teams • Office hours with low chance of having to come in when on-call as a consultant or trainee • Strong potential for academic work	• Less direct patient interaction than in some other specialties and lack of continuity of care with specialist teams often receiving the thanks of a patient and their family • Limited opportunity for private practice • Demanding specialist exams
Neurology	• An extremely cerebral specialty requiring excellent medical diagnostic skills • Few acute on-call commitments • Large potential for research with dedicated funding bodies and academic career streams	• Chronic patients with debilitating illnesses may be hard to manage • Large number of academics in post, meaning that research is often needed to secure consultant posts • Consultants may have to come in to see critically ill patients to a greater degree

Specialty	Pros	Cons
Neurosurgery	• Ability to superspecialise in a number of rapidly changing subspecialties • Extremely varied daily routine compared to some other surgical specialties • Strong potential for academic work	• Training is generally longer than for other surgical specialties • Patients may require a lot of input from physicians prior to and postoperatively, which may not be suited to all surgeons • Lack of specialist centres means that training positions within a programme can be geographically far apart
Obstetrics and gynaecology	• Good opportunity for private income • Obstetrics is often a hugely rewarding surgical specialty • Varied knowledge of both medicine and surgery is often needed	• Increased litigation (and hence medical insurance premiums) compared to other surgical specialties • Resident on-calls for specialist trainees • Emergency work can be emotionally and physically demanding
Oral and maxillofacial surgery	• Planned expansion in consultant posts • Opportunity for large private practice • Ability to provide services to more than one hospital site	• Lengthy specialist training needing medical and dental undergraduate degrees • Combined workload of NHS and private patients can be demanding • Lack of specialist centres means that training positions within a programme can be geographically far apart
Ophthalmology	• Strong potential for private practice • On-call for consultants and more junior surgeons is still often from home with minimal chance of being called in • Immediate results from some surgeries can be very rewarding	• Highly competitive specialty • Research and/or higher specialist training often required for consultant posts • Specialist exams are considered especially demanding

(Continued)

Specialty	Pros	Cons
Orthopaedics	<ul><li>Opportunity for large private practice</li><li>Interventional specialty with immediate results</li><li>Increasing use of technology may appeal to some clinicians</li></ul>	<ul><li>Competition for both training and consultant posts is currently higher than in other surgical specialties</li><li>Advent of dedicated trauma teams means some consultants may have to start being resident on call</li><li>Combined workload of NHS and private patients can be demanding</li></ul>
Palliative care	<ul><li>Can be extremely rewarding to be involved with minimising the suffering of terminally ill patients</li><li>Office hours with low chance of having to come in when on-call as a consultant</li><li>Flexible training programmes with job sharing at a senior level</li></ul>	<ul><li>Can be emotionally very challenging for both younger and more experienced clinicians</li><li>Minimal scope for private practice</li><li>Increasing administrative workload with meetings and discussions on a weekly basis</li></ul>
Plastic surgery	<ul><li>Strong potential for private practice</li><li>Cosmetic procedures are often very rewarding for the surgeon performing the operations</li><li>Good opportunities to work abroad in both developed and developing countries</li></ul>	<ul><li>Hyperspecialised field with long training needed to become a consultant</li><li>Huge competition on training posts and consultant positions – particularly in areas with lucrative private practice</li><li>Research and/or higher specialist training often required for consultant posts</li></ul>
Psychiatry	<ul><li>Office hours with low chance of having to come in when on-call as a consultant</li><li>Opportunity for some private practice</li><li>Strong links with allied health professionals is more structured than in some other specialties</li></ul>	<ul><li>Competition for both training and consultant posts is currently less than in other medical specialties with large numbers of foreign medical graduates taking specialist exams</li><li>Incorrect perception by some other clinicians that the career is less evidence-based than other specialties</li><li>Less funding for academic work</li></ul>

Specialty	Pros	Cons
Public health	• Office hours with minimal on-calls • Strong potential for academic work and teaching • Strong links with multiple specialties	• No opportunity for private practice • Increasing administrative workload with meetings and discussions on a weekly basis • Will need extra qualifications, e.g. Masters in Public Health in addition to other postgraduate exams
Radiology	• Training programmes are very well structured with less on-call commitments than in many other specialties and consultants can often report images from home out of hours • Increasing scope for interventional work with immediate results in terms of patient care • Good potential for private work	• Less follow-up of patients than in some other specialties • Postgraduate exams are generally accepted as being harder than in some other specialties • Outsourcing of reporting to hospitals overseas may have adverse effects on career outlook
Renal medicine	• Wide variety of general medicine seen in patients with renal disease • Good scope for academic research • Potential for extremely rewarding interactions with patients, who can initially be very unwell and then go on to live normal lives	• Long hours compared to some other medical specialties as dialysis patients can require complex treatment • Private practice less lucrative than some of the intervention-based specialties • Difficult sets of medical and emotional issues to deal with regarding patients on long-term renal replacement
Respiratory medicine	• Wide spectrum of acute and chronic conditions to be treated • Encompasses a large amount of general and acute medicine as part of the training and practice • Potential for interventional work is increasing as bronchoscopy starts to take over some of the roles traditionally undertaken by thoracic surgeons	• Ever-present caseload of difficult chronic patients with hard-to-treat asthma and chronic obstructive pulmonary disease (COPD) • Potential for private practice is not as great as for other more interventional specialties • Consultants may have to come in to see critically ill patients to a greater degree than other specialties

(Continued)

Specialty	Pros	Cons
Rheumatology	• Good potential for private practice • Strong tradition of basic science research as part of training programmes • An office-based specialty with minimal chance of having to go in on-call as a consultant	• Largely an outpatient specialty • Large number of academics in post, meaning that research is often needed to secure consultant posts • Few specialist-only training jobs mean that most trainees are on the general medical rota, which may not suit all
Urology	• Good opportunity for private practice • Consultants and middle-grade doctors are often on-call from home • Large variety of surgical procedures encountered on a weekly basis	• Large number of outpatient appointments and procedures compared to some other surgical specialties, which may not be suited to all • Administrative paperwork is regarded as more substantial than for hospital doctors • Some types of procedure not as rapidly changing compared to some other surgical specialties

Other specialties

There are a number of specialties not covered here, ranging from audiology to sleep medicine and allergy medicine to a career in rehabilitation. Most of these career paths are undertaken by few trainees and (with some exceptions such as transplant medicine) in general are office based with fewer on-call commitments than other specialties. Whilst they may not be under the auspices of a specific Royal College, they will all have a specialist professional body that is able to give specific advice on training issues and career paths.

Academic medicine

All medical students are given a flavour of academic medicine through the teaching provided to them in lecture halls and classrooms. In addition, some will have pursued academic degrees prior to starting medical school or during their studies in the form of an intercalated degree. Academic doctors can come from hospital medicine or general practice and typically divide up their time between clinical and academic work.

In some cases there may be an equal split during the week with 2.5 days spent on the wards and in outpatient clinic and the rest of the time spent managing a research group. Other academics may spend their time differently, e.g. perhaps just one outpatient clinic a week with the rest of the time spent purely in research.

An academic career has numerous advantages including the variety in a working week, the ability to travel and present at conferences and the understanding that, as well as treating patients, progress may be made towards understanding and treating specific conditions. There are also financial benefits, so although there may be limited time for private practice, the remuneration may be compensated for by hospital discretionary points, national career awards and links with industry, such as sitting on pharmaceutical boards, or becoming involved with biotechnology companies.

Academic doctors traditionally begin their career path by taking some time out of a training position to pursue some time in research. However, the current system allows for a number of Academic Clinical Fellows within each specialty who have a limited amount of dedicated time for research within the first few years of their training. This allows them insight into the career before deciding whether it is suitable for them.

There are many associated challenges which must be taken into consideration before pursuing an academic career. In addition to obtaining a medical degree and the necessary postgraduate qualifications, time will also need to be spent in a research institution working towards a higher degree such as an MD or a PhD. Funding for such positions is competitive and even once gained there is a constant pressure for those who continue in research and set up their own group to find further funding for consumables and for salaries for your research team as well as the continuous demand to produce high-quality publications. Although the hours at work may be less, the advent of mobile emails, instant messaging and dealing with colleagues worldwide in different time zones will often mean that the work itself pursues you at home and this needs to be taken into account for the long term when choosing such a career.

Portfolio careers

The ability to train flexibly means that it is possible to have a portfolio career, i.e. the concept of having a number of different strands to your long-term career. These strands are not necessarily equal, e.g. there may be one core aspect to your career and several non-core aspects. Each of the sums within the portfolio may be responsible for different aspects of your career.

For example, a GP may work part time for 3 days a week in his practice. This job would represent the core strand of his career and be the hub to which the other strands were linked. He may spend his fourth day attached to a local university where he is employed for 1 day a week as a communications tutor to medical students. This may involve giving lectures, small group teaching sessions and preparing end-of-term examinations. The fifth day may be spent at home with a morning where he writes both for a column in a GP magazine and produces a string of freelance articles. The afternoon may be dedicated to time spent with his two young children, whom he picks up at lunchtime from their nursery.

This concept of a portfolio means that as well as practising clinical medicine for the majority of your time, you are able to enjoy a diverse career with numerous benefits that may be both financially as well as intellectually rewarding.

Sources of further information

British Medical Journal Careers website: http://www.careers.bmj.com/
NHS careers website: http://www.nhscareers.nhs.uk/
Medical careers within the NHS: http://medicalcareers.nhs.uk/
Modernising Medical Careers: http://mmc.nhs.uk/
RemedyUK: http://www.remedyuk.net/

2

The foundation years

Key aims of this chapter

- Simplify the process of applying to foundation training
- Help with deciding on the right foundation school programme for you
- Addressing commonly asked questions about the foundation years.

Introduction

Foundation schools are deanery structures charged with managing foundation training. There are in total 25 foundation schools in the UK and they vary significantly in size; between them, overseeing anywhere between 73–812 and 67–787 F1 and F2 foundation programmes, respectively. Most foundation programmes comprise of mainly three 4-month placements, but two 6-month or 4- or 3-month combinations also exist.

It can be difficult to decide on the best foundation programme for you, but when weighing up the pros and cons of each programme, it is worth bearing in mind not only the specialty itself, but also the length of time spent in post, e.g. 3, 4 or 6 months, and the breadth of specialties available. For example, if you have already decided on a career pathway, two 6-month posts may be appropriate for you. Conversely, if you're undecided, a broader exposure to the various specialties would perhaps be more advantageous.

Available specialties

The foundation years aim to, and have the potential to, offer you a huge breadth of exposure to the various specialties in a variety of care settings, and even if you think you know which career you want to pursue, it is worth keeping your mind open to other specialties. Don't be surprised if

Table 2.1: Specialties available. Taken from Foundation Programme Annual Report 2009 UK. A number of specialties do not currently offer Foundation posts whereas in some others the split between F1 and F2 is not recorded

CCT specialty	F1	F2
Allergy	0.1%	
Anaesthetics	1.8%	0.8%
Audiological medicine	n/a	
Cardiology	4.7%	2.7%
Clinical genetics	n/a	
Clinical neurophysiology	n/a	
Clinical oncology	0.6%	1.1%
Clinical pharmacology and diabetes mellitus	0.2%	
Clinical radiology	0.2%	0.2%
Dermatology	0.1%	0.3%
Emergency medicine (Accident & Emergency)	2.2%	19.5%
Endocrinology and diabetes mellitus	3.8%	1.4%
Gastroenterology	4.9%	1.9%
General (internal) medicine	24.4%	12.3%
General practice	16.3%	
Genitourinary medicine	0.1%	0.9%
Geriatric medicine	9.4%	5.7%
Haematology	0.7%	1.1%
Immunology	n/a	
Infectious diseases	0.4%	0.3%
Intensive care medicine	2.4%	2.5%
Medical oncology	0.4%	0.6%
Medical ophthalmology	0.1%	
Neurology	0.3%	0.8%
Nuclear medicine	0.1%	0.1%
Obstetrics and gynaecology	1.4%	5.5%
Occupational medicine	0.1%	
Ophthalmology	0.1%	1.1%

CCT specialty	F1	F2
Paediatric cardiology	0.4%	
Paediatrics	2.6%	5.6%
Palliative medicine	0.4%	0.7%
Pathology: Chemical	0.2%	
Pathology: Cytogenetics and molecular genetics	n/a	
Pathology: Histopathology	0.3%	
Pathology: Medical microbiology and virology	0.5%	
Pharmaceutical medicine	n/a	
Psychiatry: Child and adolescent	n/a	
Psychiatry: Forensic	n/a	
Psychiatry: General	1.1%	4.8%
Psychiatry: Learning disability	0.1%	
Psychiatry: Old age	0.5%	
Psychiatry: Psychotherapy	n/a	
Public health medicine	0.6%	
Rehabilitation medicine	0.3%	0.5%
Renal medicine	1.2%	1.1%
Respiratory medicine	5.0%	1.7%
Rheumatology	1.0%	0.5%
Sport and exercise medicine	n/a	
Surgery: Cardiothoracic	0.6%	0.9%
Surgery: General surgery	31.4%	7.5%
Surgery: Neurosurgery	0.5%	1.0%
Surgery: Oral and maxillofacial	0.2%	
Surgery: Otolaryngology	0.4%	2.0%
Surgery: Paediatric	0.4%	0.4%
Surgery: Plastic	0.4%	0.7%
Surgery: Trauma and orthopaedic	5.6%	7.5%
Surgery: Urology	4.3%	2.1%
Tropical medicine	n/a	
Medical education	0.2%	

you find yourself on a completely different career path to the one you set out on and this may in part be influenced by life-events, which can take over and heavily influence your career.

Overall, as an F1 the greatest number of training opportunities exist in general surgery (31%), general (internal) medicine (24%) and geriatric medicine (9%). As an F2, the specialties you are exposed to are far greater and placements are available in emergency medicine (19%), general practice (16%) and general (internal) medicine (12%). In addition, more than half of all foundation schools also permit so-called specialty tasters.

Specialty tasters

Specialty tasters are usually undertaken in FY2 and comprise of no more than a 1-week 'taster' working within a different specialty, e.g. anaesthetics and critical care. These are usually left to you to organise and need to be requested through your local education provider. Most foundation schools will have a list of pre-existing tasters and with there being 59 different medical specialties to choose from the scope for a taster is vast.

The aim of a taster is to give you a snapshot of what it's like to work within a specialty you have not yet encountered, e.g. one of the smaller specialties, or in an area you may be considering entering, which either may not be quite so conventional, e.g. reproductive medicine, or on which you remain undecided. Beware, however, the quality of the experience can be highly variable and it is worthwhile talking to people who have done a taster in that area before you organise it.

Applying to a foundation programme

Application to foundation programmes occurs via a national on-line recruitment process whereby candidates apply to specific units of application (one or more foundation school) and are scored on their application form. Successful applicants are then allocated to a particular unit of application and the foundation schools are then responsible for matching you to a specific post within their school. It is worth noting that, for the purposes of the national recruitment round, some foundation schools will merge to form a single unit of application.

The vast proportion of F1 doctors are recruited following the national selection process and vacancies that arise following this process are

- Start thinking about posts and apply early
- Read the questions on the application form carefully and answer each question
- Stick to word limits and pay attention to grammar and spelling
- Answer all stems of a question for maximum points
- Do not refer to answers from other sections, as the scorer will not see the whole form or all questions
- Ask others to read your form and give constructive advice, comments, and correct typos, before you submit it
- Ensure you press 'SAVE' as you go along
- Submit your application well ahead of the application deadline, to avoid the system jams that occur last minute

Box 2.1 Tips for completing an online application form

advertised and filled locally. Importantly, for F2 there is no national process of selection, so any F2 vacancies available will be advertised and recruited for by the relevant foundation school. This is useful to consider if you've taken time out of programme.

Choosing the right foundation programme for you

There are a number of factors you should take into account when applying to a foundation programme. Type of programme, breadth and specialties exposed to and geography are often the main considerations. It is also worth trying to work out the competition for posts. Table 2.2 demonstrates the number of applicants compared to the number of vacancies. Although competition will vary from year to year, there are regions, such as Northwest Thames, South Thames, Oxford, Severn, South Yorkshire and Northern Ireland, that are consistently oversubscribed and if you are likely to score poorly it would be wise to choose and apply to less popular foundation schools, as this will increase your chance of getting your first-choice.

In addition to ranking foundation schools, once you are selected into a foundation school, you will need to rank the programmes available within that school in order of preference. The deadlines for you to complete this by will vary between foundation schools.

Table 2.2: Vacancies and number of applicants in 2007–2009. Taken from www.mmc.co.uk. For the latest figures and the details of newly created deaneries at the time of applying please consult the MMC website. Shaded boxes indicate oversubscribed deaneries

Foundation school	Vacancies 2007	Applicants 2007	Vacancies 2008	Applicants 2008	Vacancies 2009	Applicants 2009
Birmingham, Shropshire and Staffordshire	266	277	338	275	338	254
Black Country	78	46	93	90	108	92
Coventry and Warwick	85	69	90	85	87	86
East Anglia	147	163	287	214	294	215
Hereford and Worcester	66	47	73	52	75	65
Leicestershire, Northamptonshire and Rutland	130	131	152	149	143	133
Mersey	266	230	293	235	308	243
North Central Thames	306	252	340	449	315	441
North East Thames	264	257	298	321	318	441
North West Thames	306	350	263	567	270	352
North Western	485	458	537	507	536	430
North Yorkshire and East Coast	157	29	172	80	166	78
Northern	348	307	393	303	378	292
Northern Ireland	210	249	234	245	234	264
Oxford	168	291	225	241	225	245
Peninsula	148	153	198	186	196	165
Scotland	803	802	767	802	754	685
Severn	246	311	288	314	268	375
South Thames	660	773	833	978	814	964
South Yorkshire	156	178	189	207	165	213
Trent	270	246	283	237	296	201
Wales	312	315	310	283	335	298
Wessex	217	251	241	218	293	244
West Yorkshire	250	270	277	290	271	270

Academic foundation programmes

For those interested in a career in research, medical education or management, an academic foundation programme (AFP) may be for you. AFPs are programmes developed in conjunction with deaneries, NHS Academic Healthcare Trusts and universities and represent flexible pathways in which you are supported in achieving academic, teaching, or leadership and management skills through dedicated protected research time (this may be either as a 4-month block or as a day-release programme spread throughout the year) alongside achieving clinical competencies.

Approximately 5% of medical students each year will be recruited into an AFP; and in August 2009, there were 389 2-year AFPs, and a smaller number of 1-year academic programmes at both F1 and F2 level. Programmes are predominantly available in research (281), but also to a lesser extent in medical education (81) and management/leadership (15), amongst others.

AFPs are popular and if you are considering applying you should be confident in your clinical skills and be able to demonstrate academic potential, through for example, performance in exams, first-class degrees, publications as well as a commitment to academic medicine, e.g. previous research, an academic elective.

Applying for academic foundation programmes

Any final year medical student who meets the minimum person specification for recruitment to a foundation programme, with demonstrable academic potential, is eligible to apply to an AFP and the exact requirements will vary between programmes. AFPs differ immensely in terms of their focus, and when deciding on the right AFP for you, it is well worth doing your homework, i.e. ask the following questions:

- Is the emphasis of the AFP on research, education or management?
- How much time will I have allocated for clinical versus academic work?
- Does the focus of the post/research area interest me?
- Is my project clinical or lab based?
- Who is my supervisor and do they have a proven track record for supervising projects/mentoring and publishing?
- Who was the FY doctor previously in post and what was their experience of the department etc?

In addition, it is well worth visiting the department and discussing the pros and cons of the post with your potential future academic supervisor.

Importantly, most AFP posts are unbanded, so you are likely to experience a pay cut for this period of your foundation training and this may have a bearing on your decision to apply.

The application process for AFPs is separate from the main foundation programme application process. Typically, posts are advertised a year before they are due to start, so if you apply and are unsuccessful don't panic – you will not be penalised and will still have time to apply through national selection to a non-AFP.

The application forms for AFPs although similar to that in format to the application form for foundation training, will vary in the type of questions asked, which tend to centre more around your achievements, interests and career aspirations. You will also need in your application to demonstrate a clear interest in the academic field you are applying for and this may be through previous research within this field.

Frequently asked questions

Am I likely to get my foundation programme of choice?

The chance of getting your first choice of foundation programme is high, and more than 90% of applicants are allocated to their first-choice foundation school. So, when thinking about which programme to apply to ensure that it is the one you really want.

Will the medical school I graduate from restrict where I apply to?

In short, the answer to the question is 'no'. Nearly 40% of UK medical school graduates do not start foundation training in the foundation school associated to the medical school they graduated from, so the scope for movement to another region is great. Although this figure includes applicants who may not have got their first preference at their local foundation school, it is estimated that approximately one-third of applicants choose a non-local foundation school as their first choice.

Will I know where I will be working for the duration of my foundation years?

More than half (55%) of all foundation schools match applicants to fill 2-year rotations before the start of their foundation programme. Others match doctors for the first year and then may have a competitive process during the first year to match doctors to their F2 rotation.

What if I need to remain in a particular region for personal reasons?

If you are tied to a particular area for personal reasons, e.g. family, personal health or your status as prime carer for someone, you can request to be pre-allocated to a specific foundation school on these special grounds. Your application will be reviewed by a local panel and if your request is refused, there is scope to appeal. Even if you are pre-allocated to a foundation school, you will still need to submit an application and have a sufficiently high score to meet the allocation criteria for that particular school.

You may also be able to link your application to that of another person (only one) so that you will be allocated to the same foundation school, e.g. a partner or sibling. Linked applicants must rank foundation schools in the same order of preference on their application form, and the lower scoring applicant will be used to allocate both applicants to a foundation school, though not necessarily the same foundation programme.

Can I move between foundation schools once I've started a programme?

In August 2009, approximately 6% of doctors starting F2 had either transferred from a different foundation school or returned following a period out of the programme. So the scope certainly exists to transfer between foundation schools once you have been accepted onto a foundation programme. The ease at which this is achieved will be determined by both vacancies being available in your receiving foundation school and the reasons (i.e. special circumstances) for your transfer.

You will also have to demonstrate that your circumstances have changed from the time you originally applied, e.g. you are the primary carer for a disabled dependent, pregnancy, health problems etc. Any transfer will need to be approved by both the originating and receiving foundation school, but there is scope for appeal if your transfer is refused (the time allowed to appeal is however limited – typically 10 days).

Can I train flexibly?

In 2009, approximately 19 foundation schools had doctors at FY1 and FY2 level training flexibly or within supernumerary part-time posts, so yes, flexible training is very possible. You should enquire about this option early if you are considering it.

What are my chances of getting into a foundation programme as an overseas student?

In 2009 approximately 2% of FY1 doctors graduated from a medical school outside the UK, and as long as you meet the eligibility criteria, there is no reason why you shouldn't apply. Although competition is high as an overseas candidate, it is worth bearing in mind that not all foundation schools will have filled all of their posts by the start of jobs. In August 2009, 95% of FY1 places and 91% of FY2 places were filled at the start of jobs, and 2% of FY1 and 3% of FY2 places remained unfilled for the year. The reasons for not filling posts include students failing exams, resignations, failure to meet pre-employment checks and changes in circumstance.

In addition, some foundation schools have additional F1 and F2 places specifically reserved for doctors who enter the NHS with full General Medical Council (GMC) registration, but who cannot prove they have acquired competence equivalence to the foundation programme, and these posts are well worth investigating.

What if I don't want the job I'm offered or if I fail my exam?

In both cases, i.e. if you decline your job offer or fail the exam, you will be withdrawn from the application process. In the former scenario, you cannot apply for a 2-year foundation programme, as any vacancies that arise following national recruitment will typically be only for one year. In the latter case, you will need to re-apply through the same system of national recruitment the following year.

Applying to foundation courses

If you are due to qualify from a UK medical school or have qualified from a non-UK medical school and have been given approval by the UK Foundation Programme's Eligibility Office, you are eligible to apply to a foundation programme.

Details of programmes and application forms are available to view from late September; and in order to apply and view the application form you will need to register online at the official Foundation Year website. Importantly, all correspondence will be conducted via email, so you should check your email and spam mailbox regularly during this period.

Allocation to a foundation programme

You will be allocated to a foundation school based on your foundation school preferences in conjunction with your application score. Note: your overall application score is a combination of your academic score, which is based on your ranking, and your score from your application form.

Each application will in total have a maximum score of 100 points, of which 40 points is derived from your academic ranking and 60 from your application form (discussed later). Your academic ranking is calculated from your medical school results by dividing your year group into quartiles based on academic performance. Those in the first quartile (the top 25% of your year) receive a score of 40; those in the second quartile, a score of 38; those in the third quartile a score of 36 and those in the fourth quartile a score of 34.

Following selection to a foundation school, you will need to rank the foundation programmes provided by your allocated foundation school, and based on your score you will be allocated to one of these programmes. Once you are recruited to a programme, pre-employment checks will be conducted, which include Criminal Records Bureau (CRB) and occupational health checks, and you may also be required as part of this to validate answers on your application form, before you are issued with a contract from your employer.

References do not play a role in selection and are used only after foundation programmes are allocated, as part of the pre-employment check. You should ask your referee for their permission before using them, as their refusal to provide a reference will delay your employment.

The application form

The online application form consists of eight sections and is geared towards ensuring you meet the essential person specifications for foundation training (see Table 2.3). The first section contains personal information, e.g. contact information, qualifications details, a tick-box section on clinical

Table 2.3: Person specifications for foundation programmes

	Essential criteria	Demonstrated by
Eligibility	Applicants must meet the requirements set out in the Foundation Programme 2010 Eligibility Criteria	Eligibility checking
Qualifications	The applicant must have achieved, or expect to achieve, a primary medical qualification as recognised by the GMC by the start of the Foundation Programme 2010	Eligibility checking
Clinical knowledge and skills	The applicant must be familiar with and be able to demonstrate an understanding of the major principles of the GMC's *Good Medical Practice* (2006) including: ● Good clinical care ● Maintaining good medical practice ● Teaching and training, appraising and assessing ● Relationships with patients, and can apply this understanding ● Working with colleagues, and can apply this understanding ● Probity ● Health The applicant must demonstrate an understanding of the outcomes to be achieved in the Foundation Programme as set out in *The New Doctor* (2007)	Application/ pre-employment screening Clinical assessment primarily demonstrated during time at medical school and assessed by exams (where appropriate)
Language and communication skills	The applicant must have demonstrable skills in listening, reading, writing and speaking in English that enable effective communication about medical topics with patients and colleagues as set out in paragraph 22 of the GMC's *Good Medical Practice* (2006)	Application/ pre-employment screening Clinical assessment (where appropriate)
Attributes	The applicant must demonstrate: ● An understanding of the importance of the patient as the central focus of care ● The ability to prioritise tasks and information appropriately ● An understanding of the importance of working effectively with others ● The ability to communicate effectively with both colleagues and patients ● Initiative and the ability to deal effectively with pressure and/or challenge ● An understanding of the principles of equality and diversity	Application/ pre-employment screening
Probity	The applicant must demonstrate appropriate professional behaviour, i.e. integrity, honesty, confidentiality as set out in the GMC's *Good Medical Practice* (2006) The applicant must have criminal records clearance at the appropriate level subject to prevailing UK legislation	Application/ pre-employment screening

and practical skills obtained, equal opportunities information and the contact details of your two referees. The scoring panel do not have access to this section and so this information will not influence your score.

The subsequent six questions in this section are scored separately and each carries a maximum mark of 10 points. Thus, there are a total of 60 points that are derived from your application form. **Question 1** of the application form refers to academic achievements with 6 points being allocated to higher degrees and 4 points in total are awarded for other educational achievements (see Table 2.4). The first question is scored nationally and questions 2–6 are free text questions that are marked by a scoring panel.

The free-text questions are typically scored horizontally by a panel of two, of which one person is a clinician, using specific guidelines. Although each question is initially marked independently, members of the panel will finally confer to give you a final score; if there is discordance, an arbiter

Table 2.4: Points allocation in question 1 of the application form

Question 1: Part 1 (max. 6 points)	Score	Qualification or degree
	0	Primary medical qualification only
	2	An intercalated degree that does not extend the medical degree by 1 year
	3	3rd class – any type of Bachelors degree, e.g. BSc, BA
	4	2.2 class – any type of Bachelors degree, e.g. BSc, BA
	5	2.1 class – any type of Bachelors degree, e.g. BSc, BA; or a Masters degree (any class)
	6	1st class – any type of Bachelors degree, e.g. BSc, BA; or PhD
Question 1: Part 1 (max. 4 points)	**Score**	
NB: > 50% of applicants will score zero in this section, so don't panic	1	One peer-reviewed academic publication
	2	Two peer-reviewed academic publications
	1	Presentations – oral or poster presentation at national or international conference
	1	Prizes – academic/educational prizes at national level

is appointed. Importantly, panel members cannot see your response to all of the questions, only the one they are marking, so do NOT refer to your answer of another question in an answer, as the examiner will not have access to the other question or answer. Importantly, application scores cannot be appealed.

The questions in this section address certain components of the person specification and when answering these questions you need to effectively demonstrate the aspect of the person specification sought and draw upon components of *Good Medical Practice* (2006) in your answer in order to maximise your score. In addition, you must keep to the word limits and these will vary between questions.

Although the questions vary each year, below are sample questions and answers in which the applicant derived maximum points for their answers. In all questions the marker will be looking for evidence of reflective learning and/or practice and this can be achieved in the form of a structured short statement, which should include the following:

● The setting, e.g. where, people involved etc.
● What your role was, e.g. what was the aim?
● The outcome
● What aspects were done well?
● What aspects could be improved upon?
● How you would tackle the same/similar situations in the future?

Question 2 (*10 points, 250 words*)

Give two examples of specific learning needs that you identified as part of your undergraduate medical training. Compare and contrast your approaches to addressing these differing needs.

How will you use these experiences to develop your competence and performance as a foundation doctor?

Medicine requires life-long learning in order to keep up-to-date. Moreover, learning is often self-directed. The aim of this question is to gauge your ability to use reflective practice to identify deficits in your learning and to establish your motivation, commitment and attitude towards learning. It is likely that the strategies you have developed in the past will be the same ones you will use in the future and the marker is looking for evidence of critical evaluation/appraisal and your ability to identify learning opportunities and direct your learning to your needs.

I found it frustratingly difficult to reliably retain the volume of information I had covered through reading and attending lectures. I realised I better recalled facts I had actively discussed, during ward teaching for example. I emulated this process by giving peer-presentations. I structured my knowledge to communicate clearly and the ensuing questions and discussions consolidated my knowledge. Whilst alone, I practiced active recall, by testing myself with mock examination questions.

I originally found auscultation for murmurs tricky. I was uncomfortable invading patients' privacy and I felt under pressure detecting seemingly subtle signs accurately and quickly. I used textbooks and computer-controlled simulators to get a sound grasp of the theory, then discussed and observed examination technique with experienced students and doctors. Thereafter I took every opportunity to auscultate patients. I always spent time with the patient to build a rapport, gain informed consent and afterwards asked their views on my examination.

In both cases I first needed to structure the information in my mind before discussing it further with colleagues. However, in the second instance, there was no substitute for repeated experience in the clinical environment to gain competence and later proficiency.

Most importantly I realised my preferred learning style requires constant critical evaluation of my knowledge or technique be it from colleagues, patients, doctors or self-analysis. Continual professional development is integral to foundation training and I can use my identified learning techniques to reach the requisite levels of competence in clinical knowledge, practical procedures and professional skills.

Question 3 (*10 points, 250 words*)

Compare and contrast the care that you have observed for two patients with the same diagnosis and similar clinical problems. Describe the care and the extent to which it took into account the individual needs of the patients. What have you learned from these observations and how will you apply this learning to future clinical practice?

In your answer you are expected to demonstrate a clear understanding of the Duties of a Doctor as outlined in Good Medical Practice.

Patients must be able to trust doctors with their lives and health. To justify that trust you must show respect for human life and you must:

- Make the care of your patient your first concern
- Protect and promote the health of patients and the public
- Provide a good standard of practice and care
  - Keep your professional knowledge and skills up to date
  - Recognise and work within the limits of your competence
  - Work with colleagues in the ways that best serve patients' interests

- Treat patients as individuals and respect their dignity
  - Treat patients politely and considerately
  - Respect patients' right to confidentiality

- Work in partnership with patients:
  - Listen to patients and respond to their concerns and preferences
  - Give patients the information they want or need in a way they can understand
  - Respect patients' right to reach decisions with you about their treatment and care
  - Support patients in caring for themselves to improve and maintain their health

- Be honest and open and act with integrity
  - Act without delay if you have good reason to believe that you or a colleague may be putting patients at risk
  - Never discriminate unfairly against patients or colleagues
  - Never abuse your patients' trust in you or the public's trust in the profession

Box 2.2 Duties of a doctor registered with the General Medical Council (*Good Medical Practice*, 2009)

Answer

Whilst observing in the GP clinic, I encountered two heavy smokers with type 2 diabetes. Both were poorly compliant with similar medication regimens leaving them with persistently high blood sugar. The first, an elderly man with a supportive wife, now suffered leg pain likely related to diabetic complications. The second, a middle-aged woman, was still asymptomatic but under much stress through having to look after her recently disabled husband. The initial aim for both was to encourage smoking cessation and improve compliance.

The man's co-morbidity made stopping smoking the priority. Though previously resistant he became amenable once he understood smoking worsened symptoms and rendered other treatments less effective. The GP recruited the man's wife and the 'Stop Smoking' Nurse so the couple could stop together and support each other through the process.

In contrast, the second patient had a poor support network and used smoking to cope. She felt quitting would cause greater problems at this stage. The GP therefore focussed on compliance, explaining the relevance of diabetes and role of medication. Together they devised coping strategies that allowed her time to put her own health first, leaving the option to quit available for the future.

This experience showed me the importance of respecting patient choice and taking a holistic approach to healthcare through considering their physical, psychological and social needs. During foundation training this will help me develop effective relationships with patients and share decision making with them so that they can more easily take ownership of their treatment plans.

Question 4 (*8 points, 150 words*)

Describe one example of a clinical situation where you demonstrated or observed appropriate professional behaviour despite difficult circumstances. How will you apply what you have learned to your future practice?

The focus of this question is the doctor–patient partnership. Good Medical Practice *states that the doctor–patient relationship is "based on openness, trust and good communication (and this) will enable you to work in partnership with your patients to address their individual needs (see Box 2.2)." In answering this question, you should think of a scenario, e.g. breaking bad news, where aspects of the relationship were met or perhaps not met, and in your answer you should demonstrate empathy and sympathy.*

The doctor–patient partnership (*Good Medical Practice*, 2009)

To fulfil your role in the doctor–patient partnership you must:

- Be polite, considerate and honest
- Treat patients with dignity
- Treat each patient as an individual

- Respect patients' privacy and right to confidentiality
- Support patients in caring for themselves to improve and maintain their health
- Encourage patients who have knowledge about their condition to use this when they are making decisions about their care.

To communicate effectively you must:

- Listen to patients, ask for and respect their views about their health, and respond to their concerns and preferences
- Share with patients, in a way they can understand, the information they want or need to know about their condition, its likely progression, and the treatment options available to them, including associated risks and uncertainties
- Respond to patients' questions and keep them informed about the progress of their care
- Make sure that patients are informed about how information is shared within teams and among those who will be providing their care
- Make sure, wherever practical, that arrangements are made to meet patients' language and communication needs.

Answer

During a general medical attachment I saw a middle-aged-man with breathlessness. I accompanied him for investigations daily and we developed a good relationship. Sadly, findings suggested lung cancer with a poor prognosis. Days later the results had still not been communicated to him.

He felt anxious, overlooked and unable to approach his doctors. He asked if I would tell him his diagnosis. I would have been out of my depth conveying this news but felt dishonest withholding it.

I apologised for his distress, resisted disclosing further details, but undertook the responsibility of acting as his advocate. I alerted the registrar and stayed with the patient whilst the bad news was delivered.

I learned to handle difficult situations with a clear head, find solutions proactively and seek help when tasks were beyond my capabilities. Despite the time pressures of foundation training this approach will allow me to maintain honesty and good professional relationships.

Question 5 (*8 points, 150 words*)

Describe one example, not necessarily clinical, that has increased your understanding of team working. Describe your role and how you contributed to the team. What have you learned and how will you apply this to working with colleagues as a foundation doctor?

The factors required for good team working are outlined in the GMC's document Good Medical Practice *(2006). In general, good team working relies on ensuring that:*

- *The skills and contributions of each member of the team are respected*
- *You listen to and take on board each team member's views*
- *Communication is effective both within as well as outside the team*
- *Each member of the team understands their own role as well the role of every other member of the team*
- *The team's performance is regularly reviewed and any areas for improvement are identified and addressed*
- *Support is given to team members who are in need/distress.*

Your answer should once again be personal to you and you should try and draw upon the various components mentioned earlier. Note the use of 'we' and 'together' in the example answer given below.

Answer

Wilderness medicine is healthcare in austere or remote environments. In 2006 I co-founded UCL Wilderness Medical Society and was later elected President. Together our committee organised talks and workshops by international experts. Since its inception it has become one of the largest groups of its kind in the country.

I chaired regular planning meetings, where I encouraged open communication and valued the contributions of all team members. I maximised efficiency by identifying team members' individual strengths, assigning roles and delegating tasks accordingly.

I regularly invited feedback, consequently learning the importance of flexibility and reallocation of resources if team members needed further support. Though it was difficult when there were disparate views, I remained focussed on our goals and sought to negotiate effective compromise.

During foundation training these experiences will leave me better able to respect, communicate and work with other multiprofessional team members to reach our objectives together.

Question 6 (*8 points, 150 words*)

Describe a situation, not necessarily clinical, where you personally felt challenged and under pressure. Describe how you responded. What did you learn from this experience and how will this benefit you as a foundation doctor?

This is an example of a behavioural or situational question. Behavioural or situational questions are becoming increasingly popular in medicine and are used to assess your performance in the past, the theory being that past performance is often the best predictor of future performance in a similar situation.

Situational questions typically require you to demonstrate one key person specific quality, in this case your ability to act under pressure. Importantly, your answer should be specific and incorporate some background/scene-setting information (this should be brief), the specific action you took (which demonstrates a specific quality within the person specification) and the positive outcome. You should use 'real' personal examples, and most of all avoid embellishing the truth or exaggerating, as any experienced marker will easily spot this.

Answer

The period preceding my snowboarding instructor exams was stressful because I had to push myself to reach the high level of skill required. I took responsibility for my training, identified my weaknesses and designed a schedule that prioritised them. With a few weeks left, I suffered an injury and began struggling.

After discussion with my mentor I focussed on the teaching component, which was not as physically challenging. I also recruited other trainees to help with my learning. Though I had to postpone the technical component, I passed the teaching exam.

Initially I was failing because I had not properly acknowledged the different circumstances when moving from the practical lessons to the classroom. Later I became realistic and learned to re-prioritise, thus achieving a satisfactory outcome, despite the setback I had encountered.

Foundation training has many time pressures and I have learned to organise myself, reorganise and persevere. I will also endeavour to recognise demands placed on colleagues and help with the redistribution of workload when appropriate.

Question 7 (*8 points, 150 words*)

Describe one of your non-academic achievements. Explain clearly why this was an achievement for you. What did you learn from this achievement and how will this influence your approach to patient care?

Once again this question asks you to use reflective practice to draw on components of the person specification, e.g. teamwork, good communication, professionalism, critical appraisal etc., taken from a context outside medicine. The question also looks for a life outside medicine, i.e. are you well-rounded? It is therefore essential that the example you give is not medical or academic, otherwise you will score poorly.

Answer

I recently qualified as a Divemaster following months of dedicated training to ensure I could manage recreational divers and take responsibility for their safety when leading dives and assisting instruction. Divemasters are role models and I had to demonstrate professional standards of competence and conduct. Very few divers make this transition to professional level.

Diving is potentially extremely dangerous and I have learned extended rescue management and problem-solving skills to cope. I know it is imperative to seek help from senior colleagues in serious situations, but ultimately I realised the need for teamwork and communication to prevent problems arising from the outset.

There are many parallels between being a Divemaster and a foundation doctor beyond maintaining safety and professionalism. I am considerate of divers' needs, encourage and support them as well as make decisions together with them. I intend to bring all these skills to my approach to patient care.

Sources of further information

NHS Foundation Programme: http://www.foundationprogramme.nhs.uk
Modernising Medical Careers: http://www.mmc.nhs.uk
NHS foundation support: http://www.nhscareers.nhs.uk/foundationtraining

3

Getting through the foundation years

Key aims of this chapter

- Give an understanding of the forms of assessment used within the foundation years
- Give an overview of the foundation curriculum
- Advise on how to get the most from your foundation programme.

Introduction

The foundation programme was introduced in August 2005, and intends to give the trainee a structured, well-supervised competency-based approach to training. It spans a 2-year period (usually commencing in August) and is composed of placements of between 3–6 months in length (predominantly 4 months) within various specialties. Foundation training in essence is the bridge between medical school and core, specialty, and GP training.

As an FY1/FY2 (F1/F2) doctor you will be continually assessed against standards set out in the Foundation Programme Curriculum (June 2007) and are required to maintain a portfolio of achievements that demonstrates your competencies.

Importantly, your portfolio will remain with you throughout training and most likely through the duration of your medical career. The aim of this chapter is to give you an idea of what to expect as a FY doctor, what is expected of you and ways in which you can maximise your training opportunities and get the most from your clinical experiences.

- Highlight achievements and areas of excellence
- Emphasise the need for feedback
- Supply and demonstrate evidence of progression linked to the Curriculum
- Identify doctors who may need additional help

The Foundation Programme Curriculum (the Curriculum) sets out the framework for educational progression that will support the first 2 years of professional development after graduation from medical school .... The Curriculum separates out F1 and F2 competences and is based on *Good Medical Practice* (2006)

Box 3.1 Purpose of assessment as defined in Foundation Curriculum

All medical graduates are required to complete a 2-year foundation programme in order to practice as a doctor in the UK. Once you have successfully completed FY1, through achievement of the necessary competencies, you can not only apply for full registration with the GMC, but also progress into FY2. Following completion of FY2, you will receive a Foundation Achievement of Competence Document (FACD) – this is a prerequisite for entry into specialty training.

Before you start work, you will need to be provisionally registered with the GMC. As an F1 the GMC has overall responsibility for your training and in subsequent years, the Postgraduate Medical Education and Training Board (PMETB) will take on this role and is responsible for setting training standards as described below:

1.0 Professionalism

    1.1 Behaviour in the workplace
    1.2 Health and handling stress and fatigue
    1.3 Time management and continuity of care.

2.0 Good clinical care

    2.1 Eliciting a history
    2.2 Examination
    2.3 Diagnosis and clinical decision making
    2.4 Safe prescribing
    2.5 Medical record keeping and correspondence
    2.6 Safe use of medical devices.

3.0 Recognition and management of the acutely ill patient

3.1 Promptly assessesing the acutely ill or collapsed patient

3.2 Identifying and responding to acutely abnormal physiology

3.3 Where appropriate, delivering a fluid challenge safely to an acutely ill patient

3.4 Reassessing ill patients appropriately after starting treatment

3.5 Undertaking a further patient review to establish a differential diagnosis

3.6 Obtaining an arterial blood gas sample safely, and interpreting results correctly

3.7 Managing patients with impaired consciousness, including those with convulsions

3.8 Using common analgesic drugs safely and effectively

3.9 Understanding and applying the principles of managing a patient with an acute mental disorder

3.10 Ensuring safe continuing care of patients on handover between shifts, on-call staff or with 'hospital at night' team.

4.0 Resuscitation

4.1 Resuscitation

4.2 Discussing Do Not Attempt Resuscitation (DNAR) orders/advance directives appropriately.

5.0 Discharge and planning for chronic disease management

6.0 Relationship with patients and communication skills

6.1 Within a consultation

6.2 Breaking bad news.

7.0 Patient safety within clinical governance

7.1 Treating the patient as the centre of care

7.2 Making patient safety a priority in own clinical practice

7.3 Promoting patient safety through good team working

7.4 Understanding the principles of quality and safety improvement

7.5 Complaints.

8.0 Infection control

9.0 Nutritional care

10.0 Health promotion, patient education and public health

10.1 Educating patients
10.2 Environmental, biological and lifestyle risk factors
10.3 Smoking
10.4 Alcohol
10.5 Epidemiology and screening.

11.0 Ethical and legal issues

11.1 Medical ethical principles and confidentiality
11.2 Valid consent
11.3 Legal framework of medical practice
11.4 Relevance of outside bodies.

12.0 Maintaining good medical practice

12.1 Lifelong learning
12.2 Research, evidence, guidelines and care protocols
12.3 Audit.

13.0 Teaching and training

14.0 Working with colleagues

14.1 Communication with colleagues and teamwork for patient safety
14.2 Interface with different specialties and with other professionals.

At the start of each placement, you should receive an induction in addition to information about the workplace, rota, and an outline of your responsibilities; you should also be given the name of your educational supervisor.

All F1 and F2 doctors will have a named educational supervisor allocated to them at the beginning of their post. Your educational supervisor (usually a senior doctor) is there to support your educational needs throughout your training programme and is responsible for helping you meet your educational agreement and this may be through:

● Supervising your day-to-day clinical activity
● Ensuring you are able to meet educational sessions, e.g. bleep-free teaching

- Providing support and guidance regarding assessments and developing your learning portfolio
- Ensuring you have a good mix in terms of clinical exposure
- Acting as a point of contact for concerns regarding training.

Preparing your portfolio

Under *Modernising Medical Careers* the emphasis is on achieving competencies. A logbook of procedures/operations and references on their own are no longer sufficient and applicants are expected to provide proof of their educational activities and professional development in the form of a portfolio.

Components of a portfolio

Portfolios were initially developed in the 1940s and have been popular as a tool for assessing professional competence and proficiency in occupations such as architecture and the arts for some time. It has however not been until recently that they have become popular in medicine.

Owing to their flexible nature and multiple components portfolios are thought to give a more representative view of you as an individual than perhaps your CV alone. However, your portfolio is only as good as you make it, and the more effort you put into it, the more you will get out of it.

In addition to its use as a selection tool for specialty training, your portfolio should encourage you to reflect upon your achievements, identify your strengths and weaknesses and help you to direct your future learning,

---

- Allocate time each month to updating your portfolio
- Ensure assessments are evenly spaced throughout the programme so progress can be more clearly evidenced
- Look out for training and learning opportunities; you are responsible for your learning and should not expect to be spoon-fed
- Identify and target deficiencies in your training early
- If you are having problems getting assessments completed, it may prove easier to print out blank paper assessment forms for your assessor to complete

Box 3.2 Tips on completing your portfolio

i.e. it should encourage reflective learning and facilitate continued professional development (CPD).

Most foundation schools have online so-called e-portfolios for trainees. The completed e-portfolio will not only contribute to the end-of-year report – it may also be used in interviews. Your foundation portfolio should include:

- A list of competencies required to successfully complete the foundation programme
- Records of meetings with your educational supervisor
- A personal development plan (PDP) including career planning.

Presented evidence

- Exam certificates
- Certificates of course/lecture/tutorial attendance
- Posters presented at learned meetings
- Presentations including at journal clubs
- Abstracts and papers (full texts)
- Audit projects (full texts)
- A reflective log of activities and experience
- A logbook of clinical activity or record of achieved competencies signed by your trainer, e.g. procedures or operations.

Workplace-based assessments (WBAs)

- 360-degree assessments or mini-peer assessment tools (mini-PATs)
- Directly observed procedures (DOPs)
- Mini-clinical evaluation exercise (mini-CEX)
- Case-based discussions (CBDs)
- Procedure-based assessments (PBAs).

Developing your portfolio

You are responsible for your own learning, ensuring your assessments are completed, and keeping your portfolio kept up-to-date. Throughout foundation training (and indeed your career), each clinical encounter should be treated as a learning opportunity and your portfolio should demonstrate progression of your skills throughout the year, your achievements and reflective practice. Importantly, you will not be signed off for foundation training, without a satisfactory portfolio and to get the most from your portfolio, you should organise a regular review of your portfolio with your educational supervisor.

The number and type of assessment that needs to be performed will vary and be determined by your foundation school. They will also inform you about the deadline for their submission. Importantly, do not leave completion of your assessments until the last placement, as it is likely that your colleagues who you are asking to complete them will be bombarded with several other requests and may not be so keen to act as an assessor.

Workplace assessments

Workplace-based assessments (WBAs) form an integral part of assessment of competency for foundation trainees. The tools used are formative, and therefore are designed to give constructive feedback, which not only ensures that a trainee continually improves their practice and progresses satisfactorily but also provides documented evidence of their learning and development. Moreover, these type of assessments can be used to identify any problems you may be experiencing early and in addition provide constructive feedback that will focus and guide your further personal development. Importantly, these assessments will inform your educational supervisor's report to the deanery and this will influence whether you are recommended for full GMC registration at the end of F1.

The principles for assessment and guidance on WBAs are established by the Postgraduate Medical Education Training Board (PMETB).

WBA is a term that embraces a spectrum of assessment tools including: 360-degree assessments or mini-PAT; mini-CEX; DOPs; case-based discussions (CBDs) and procedure-based assessments (PBAs). The underlying principle is that trainees are assessed on work that they actually perform and thus the assessment is integrated into the trainees day-to-day work. For WBA to be effective the method of assessment must be robust (quality assured), reliable, valid and fit for purpose and trainees should:

- Understand the purpose of the assessment
- Be given formative feedback following assessment that will inform and guide their personal development
- Be assessed by a number of different assessors or trainers
- Be assessed over a broad range of activities, using a number of different 'assessment tools', e.g. foundation trainees are expected to undertake a minimum of 20 assessments.

Work-based assessment is 'trainee led' and it is up to the trainee to identify suitable opportunities and decide when, where and who will assess them, with the guidance of their educational supervisor. Anyone competent in performing the assessed competency may act as an assessor. Each encounter should typically take 15 minutes and a further 5 minutes is then devoted to meaningful formative feedback. Each assessment is scored using a structured ticklist form and a copy is held by the trainee as part of the body of evidence of satisfactory progression contained within the trainee's (electronic) learning portfolio; this portfolio will be subject to an annual review.

It is worth bearing in mind that you will be assessed against the standard of competence that is expected of a doctor completing the F1/F2 training. If, initially, you don't meet the required standard, do not be disheartened as this will not count against you, as long as by the end of the year you have progressed to the required competency level.

Types of workplace assessment

360-degree assessments, mini-peer assessment tool or multi-source feedback

The 360-degree assessment otherwise known as the mini-PAT or multi-source feedback (MSF) is a concept that originated from the commercial sector and is a process whereby evidence regarding your performance at work is gathered from a number of different co-workers. The list should be agreed with your educational supervisor and may include medical colleagues (of different grades), your educational supervisor, non-medical members of your team, e.g. secretarial or clerical staff, biomedical scientists, nurses, pharmacists etc. In some specialties it may be appropriate to involve patients. The theory is that by taking a 'multi-source' approach, a more holistic and objective view of you as a doctor within a team-working environment can be achieved. 360-degree assessments are thought to be more fair compared to the traditional single-source reference, which has the potential to be open to bias.

Methods that can be used in formal 360-degree appraisal may include unstructured interviews, statements with a simple rating scale and more commonly, structured questionnaires using indicators of good performance, as determined by *Good Medical Practice*. Once sufficient responses are received, the information is gathered, analysed and the results constructively fed back anonymously to the appraisee/trainee by the trainee's educational supervisor and used to guide their personal development.

- Should be undertaken in the first 4 months of the year and repeated in the last 4 months of training if concerns are raised
- 15 raters should be nominated
- A minimum of 10 returns are required for assessment
- NB: No other foundation doctor can be a rater
- The recommended mix of raters/assessors is:
  - 2–8 doctors more senior than F2, including at least one consultant or GP principal
  - 2–6 senior nurses (band 5 or above)
  - 2–4 allied health professionals
  - 2–4 other team members including ward clerks, secretaries and auxiliary staff

Box 3.3 Recommendations for multi-source feedback

For the purposes of your portfolio, in addition to your mini-PAT, you could include additional 'multi-source' evidence in the form of thank you letters from patients or letters recognising your contribution to aspects of your working life, e.g. mess president, rota development etc.

Mini clinical evaluation exercise

The mini-CEX is a method of assessing professional skills such as history taking, physical examination, clinical judgement, communicating results or discussing management with patients, professionalism, presentation skills, involvement in MDT (Multi Disciplinary Meeting) meetings and others skills essential for good clinical care, as determined by the specialty-specific curriculum within the work setting.

Assessors do not need to have prior knowledge of the trainee, however should be competent in the area being assessed. Their evaluation is recorded on a structured checklist and constructive verbal feedback is given to the trainee immediately following the assessment/encounter. The whole process should take between 15–20 minutes.

Directly observed procedures

DOPs is a concept initially developed by the UK Royal College of Physicians that aims to assess competency, i.e. ability whilst performing a practical skill or part or all of a practical procedure within the work setting, e.g. on

- A minimum of six mini-CEX in F1 and another six in F2 should be completed
- Assessments should be evenly spaced out during the year
- >2 mini-CEX should be completed in each 4-month period
- A different assessor should ideally be used for each mini-CEX including:
  - at least one of consultant or GP level, per 4-month placement
- Each mini-CEX must represent a different clinical problem

Box 3.4 Guidelines for mini-CEX

the ward, in outpatients, or in theatre. The practical competencies assessed will be determined by the trainees' level and also their specialty. For example, at foundation level, index competencies listed on the curriculum include venesection, cannulation, blood culture, urethral catheterisation and intubation, amongst others.

The process of assessment should typically take between 15–20 minutes. The assessors can be any healthcare professional (e.g. specialist registrar [SpR] nurse, consultant, or pharmacist) competent in performing the assessed skill and they do not necessarily have to have prior knowledge of the trainee.

Following performance of the task the assessor should give the trainee immediate feedback and their evaluation is documented on a structured checklist form, which is returned to the trainee and a copy is retained for the trainee's portfolio. It is your responsibility to arrange the assessments and submit copies of the reports.

- Up to three DOPs can be submitted as part of the minimum requirements for evidence assessing doctor–patient encounters
- Different assessors should ideally be used for each encounter
- Each DOP could represent a different procedure and may be specific to the specialty
- DOPs can be used in foundation training to assess the doctor–patient interaction

Box 3.5 Guidelines for DOPs

Case-based discussions

A CBD is a structured in-depth interview, designed to assess a trainee's clinical judgment, decision-making skill, ability to prioritise and application of medical knowledge, through discussion of a challenging clinical case managed by the trainee. This should include a detailed discussion of the actions taken, as well as any ethical and legal considerations, e.g. record keeping.

The CBD tool can be applied to both hospital and GP settings and the assessor should be a senior colleague, e.g. a GP trainer, SpR or consultant. Assessments should take between 15–20 minutes and following completion of the assessment form (which may only be performed online), immediate and structured feedback should be given, which would normally take about 5 minutes. CBD essentially formalises a well-established practice of presenting and discussing clinical cases by trainees and couples it with formal feedback. At foundation level the criteria for assessment includes: (1) medical record keeping; (2) clinical assessment; (3) investigations and referrals; (4) treatment; (5) follow-up and future planning; (6) professionalism and (7) overall clinical judgment.

- A minimum of six CBDs should be completed
- At least two CBDs should be performed in any 4-month period
- Where possible, different assessors should be used for each CBD
- Assessors should have sufficient experience in the area assessed, e.g. specialty training
- Each CBD must tackle a different clinical problem

Box 3.6 Guidelines for CBDs

Procedure-based assessment

PBA is a tool that is not dissimilar from DOPs, however, it is specific to the surgical specialties. The aim of PBA is to assess the 'technical ability and professional skills' of the trainee in a range of index procedures or parts of procedures, as appropriate to the level of the trainee. The assessor following the procedure, using an assessment form that outlines both the desirable and undesirable behaviours, will be required to provide the trainee with constructive feedback that will guide future practice. The ultimate standard is that achieved for Certificate of Completion of Training (CCT).

Reflective log of activities and experience

Reflective practice is a concept that was initially coined in the 1980s by Donald Schön and is defined as a continuous process that involves "thoughtfully considering one's own experiences in applying knowledge to practice while being coached by professionals in the discipline".

In essence, reflective practice can be seen as a form of experiential learning. It requires the analysis of past experiences or performances, critique of these events with the identification of aspects that were done well, as well as those that could be improved upon, with the aim of adapting your approach for future situations. The process of reflection can occur 'in action', i.e. immediately – whilst performing the task or 'on action', i.e. at a later stage.

Within your portfolio you should be able to demonstrate reflective learning and/or practice and this can be achieved in the form of a structured short statement. This should include the following:

● The setting, e.g. where, people involved etc.
● Your role
● The outcome
● Aspects done well
● Aspects that could be improved upon
● How you would tackle the same or similar situations in the future.

If you need help with developing your portfolio, points of contact include:

● Your educational supervisor
● Your foundation school
● Your local foundation programme tutor/director.

Your personal development plan or educational agreement

A PDP identifies your learning needs and sets time-limited goals on how these may be met and demonstrated. Learning needs can be identified by drawing upon the Foundation Programme Curriculum (June 2007) and through discussions with your educational supervisor. However, you may yourself identify clear gaps in your knowledge or experience, and there are a number of teaching and learning tools you can engage to address this; these may include:

● Courses
● E-learning modules

- Simulators
- Use of skills laboratory facilities
- Audit
- Team discussions
- Patient encounters.

The Foundation programme is the platform from which you will enter specialty training, however application and recruitment into core, specialty, or GP training posts will occur whilst you are partway through F2. You should start to think about the specialty you want to pursue early, and your PDP should include aims that involve meeting the person specification for your desired career pathway. This may include sitting postgraduate exams, embarking on research, conducting audit projects, developing courses, teaching and attending specific courses, e.g. ALS, ATLS (you will not be eligible for study leave or money as an F1).

To gain the most from your training, you should aim to meet your educational and clinical supervisor (these may be the same people) at the start of your post and at regular intervals throughout your foundation programme; the onus is on you to organise these meetings.

The initial meeting or appraisal should include discussion regarding learning opportunities available, areas of interest to you, potential areas for improvement or weaknesses and a discussion of your strengths. An educational agreement should be drawn at this initial meeting, with discussion of timelines and methods through which your needs contained within the agreement can be met.

At the end of each post, you will be required to meet with your educational supervisor for an overall review of your progress within a particular placement and part of this final appraisal will include evaluation of your e-portfolio, i.e. the results of assessments made during the placement, observations from colleagues and other members of your team etc. This meeting will conclude with the completion of a 'sign off' document, which will confirm satisfactory performance and progress, and/or highlight outstanding concerns/issues. The outcome of the final assessment discussion has to be agreed by both parties (so if you feel unfairly viewed, there is scope for discussion) and is recorded in your e-portfolio on the 'end of placement review' form. These individual placement reports together will form part of the body of evidence given for recommendation of satisfactory completion of F1, and subsequently, the foundation programme.

Foundation year 2

Following successful progression in FY1, most doctors will progress seamlessly into FY2. Some foundation schools have a process of competitive entry from FY1 to FY2, and although you are guaranteed an FY2 post if this occurs, it may not be in your desired specialties. Other foundation schools will allocate FY2 jobs based on the preferences you've given at the time of the first application.

The range of specialties encountered at FY2, is far greater than that within FY1 and you will also have the opportunity to experience areas such as general practice and undertake so-called 'tasters' (periods of no more than 1 week), within a specialty you may be interested in.

As an FY2 doctor, you will be subject to the same assessment processes as an FY1, however, the standard of competencies will differ. In a similar manner, you will need to maintain an up-to-date portfolio, which will be used to inform the postgraduate dean of your satisfactory progress in FY2.

Making the most of FY2 placement in general practice

There are broadly three types of FY2 doctors doing a GP FY2 placement: those who wish to be GPs, those who do not, and those who are undecided.

The benefits of an FY2 placement for those who are considering general practice are self-evident. This is an opportunity to sample a career in a relatively protected setting and yet you can see patients alone, visit patients alone, and instigate investigations and management plans. All of these will be reviewed by a clinical supervisor. By doing a placement in general practice, FY2 doctors also get a glimpse of what the Royal College of General Practitioners (RCGP) curriculum and e-portfolio hold in store, should they pursue a career as a GP.

The RCGP e-portfolio is matched to the curriculum and links to particular competencies. Multi-source feedback, DOPs, and CBD continue to be used as forms of work-based assessment. GP placements also use a consultation observation tool (COT), where an appraiser/assessor sits in with or watches a video of a trainee while they consult. Whilst videos are not compulsory, they are a good way for trainees to see what they actually do say and do. Access to these types of resources are generally something not available in other types of FY2 placement.

FY2 doctors who are sure they do not wish to follow a career in general practice are presented with an opportunity to understand what is available in the community, how undifferentiated problems are filtered into a referral, and how problems are managed outside the hospital environment. It is particularly useful to understand what it is like to be on the other end of a referral to secondary care. The importance of discharge planning and even a prompt and properly written discharge letter finds new emphasis. Moreover, this may also be the last time that some types of problems are encountered on a regular basis, such as psychiatry, paediatrics and gynaecology.

Rather than ignoring these types of patient as 'irrelevant' (for example) to a career in surgery, a placement in general practice is an opportunity to improve and retain some skills that may come in handy for the future. General practice is also an excellent environment for learning essential skills that are sometimes perceived as softer, such as communication and time-management skills. In addition, there are also opportunities to do courses in and even to practice (usually under supervision) minor surgery. Minor surgery courses are run by the RCGP and the RSM, as well as other educational bodies and commercial companies. These are extremely popular with GP trainees and new GPs, so it is worth bearing in mind that they do get booked up extremely quickly.

Having the right attitude to a placement may also make a huge difference to the benefits derived from a placement and how functional the relationship is with your trainer/clinical supervisor. Those with aspirations towards community paediatrics, whether as a paediatrician or a GP, may consider doing the Diploma in Child Health, which no longer requires a formal paediatric placement. Other postgraduate diplomas that may be considered include the Diploma of the Royal College of Obstetricians and Gynaecologists or the Diploma in Geriatrics.

If considering these options, bear in mind the lead time needed to book into exams and to revise or attend courses. For example FY2 trainees considering the Diploma in Child Health (DCH) exam should consider doing the multiple choice question (MCQ paper) before their placement in paediatrics or general practice so they have the knowledge and time to book (and practice for) the objective structured clinical examination (OSCE). Courses and exam slots get booked up quickly, and candidates may have to consider attending a more distant centre or planning ahead.

Frequently asked questions

Am I entitled to study leave?

Although as an FY1 doctor you are not entitled to study leave per se, your foundation training programme director (FTPD) should ensure you receive formal protected, i.e. bleep-free, teaching.

In F2, you are eligible for 30 days' study leave per year, and you should use this wisely. If you are training flexibly, you are still entitled to the full study budget allocation; however, the time for study leave will be calculated based on your hours of training. Study leave is not required to sit specialist examinations (see chapter 8 for more details).

In general, it is worthwhile spending both your leave and study budget as an F2 on:

- A specific required course, e.g. ALS, ATLS, or Basic Surgical Skills
- Courses that may enhance your communication or teaching skills
- Accessing simulators.

Where can I go for careers advice?

You need to actively think about the career path you wish to pursue during your foundation year. Moreover, if undecided your PDP can be used to increase your exposure to as many specialties as possible, e.g. through 'tasters'. It is worthwhile writing a list of your values, strengths and weaknesses, or likes and dislikes in medicine, and try to match it with the skills, attitudes etc. required for various career options.

When deciding upon a career, you should also have a realistic idea of where you stand amongst the competition, and consider future job prospects within that given area. Your e-portfolio will form the centre point for any discussion around careers, and there are a number of avenues that you can pursue for careers counselling/advice, including:

- Your educational or clinical supervisor
- Your FTPD (this is an individual appointed by the deanery and trust to manage and lead a foundation training programme)
- Careers fairs
- Senior colleagues
- The deanery/foundation school – they should have a dedicated careers service
- The relevant Royal College and specialty clinical tutors

- Publications, e.g. *BMJ Careers*
- UK Medical Careers website www.medicalcareers.nhs.uk.

It is well worth trying to engage and have on board a senior doctor within your specialty of interest as a mentor early, and often they will prove to be an invaluable source of advice throughout your career.

Once you have a career/specialty in mind, and even if you haven't, there are a number of things you can do to put yourself ahead of the competition. This may be in the form of:

- Postgraduate exams – these are being undertaken at foundation year
- Specialty specific courses, e.g. in basic laparoscopic skills
- Audit
- Research projects within your field of interest.

Can I defer my start date on a foundation programme?

Following discussion and agreement with your educational supervisor, and on acceptable grounds, it is possible to defer the start of your programme once you have been accepted onto a 2-year programme, and this typically will not be for any longer than 1 year. You should however give adequate (usually more than 3 months) notice.

Can I train flexibly?

There are a number of reasons why you may want to train flexibly, e.g. children, personal health, work–life balance, life events etc., and there are established mechanisms in place through which you can apply for flexible training. Although you do not need to state your intention to train flexibly when you apply for foundation training, it is worthwhile discussing your intention to train flexibly early with the deanery, in order for them to assess your eligibility and allow them time to accommodate your needs. In order to comply with the requirements of the European Specialist Qualification Order (1995) as a flexible trainee you must undertake training on at least a half-time basis. In certain circumstances, you may be supernumerary within a post.

Can I transfer between deaneries/foundation schools?

The scope certainly exists to transfer between foundation schools once you have been accepted onto a foundation programme. The ease at which this is achieved however will be determined by both vacancies being available in your receiving foundation school and the reasons (i.e. special circumstances) for your transfer. You will also have to demonstrate that your circumstances have changed, e.g. you are the primary carer for a disabled dependent, pregnancy, health problems etc., from the time you originally applied. Transfers usually occur at the start of F1 or F2, but you can apply for transfer at any time. Any transfer will need to be approved by both the originating and receiving foundation school, but there is scope for appeal if your transfer is refused.

Can I train abroad?

Providing that the post is approved prospectively for training by the postgraduate deanery, it is possible to spend your F2 year abroad. The emphasis is on you, however, to identify a suitable programme, seek training approval and ensure assessments are conducted by your host institution. Countries commonly worked in include Australia, New Zealand and America.

Can I take time out?

This is possible, and if you are considering this as an option, you should discuss it with your educational supervisor or foundation programme training director (FPTD). You will need to have a good reason for taking time out and will need to complete a Time Out of Foundation Programme (TOFP) proforma (obtained from your FPTD), and this should be completed in the first 6 months of training, where possible. Time-out is usually for 1 year, though shorter time blocks may be an option depending on your circumstances.

Importantly, you need to inform your FPTD of your intention to return to the programme 6 months before the start of your placement.

Do doctors fail to complete the foundation programme?

Approximately 98% of F1 and 96% of F2 doctors in 2009 successfully completed their foundation years and were signed off as having attained the appropriate level of competence. Reasons for not completing F1/F2 included having more than 4 weeks' absence, with a requirement for remedial training, being dismissed and resigning. Out of the total of F1 doctors from UK medical schools, 5% required additional support versus 41% of graduates from non-UK medical schools. In addition, in 2009, eight F1 doctors and nine F2 doctors were referred to the GMC for fitness to practice issues.

Who can I turn to for help?

Things can go wrong and if this occurs you should raise the issue early and not be afraid to do so. There is help and support available, even if you feel nobody can help. The competency assessment process is designed to ensure that any problems are flagged up early and this may be through recognition of the problem by you or by others, failure to progress etc. Strategies are available that can be employed to resolve the problem as soon as possible, at every stage of your training, for example, more focussed training.

Your educational supervisor should be your first port of call, and should be able to guide you in the right direction. Alternatively, you can speak to the FPTD.

What if I fail?

If you are not be able to demonstrate the required level of competence in the first year, you will not be granted full registration with the GMC and will not be able to progress to F2. You will, however, be given remedial support for up to 1 additional year. If, following this time you still have not met the required standards, you would not be allowed to practise medicine.

Should you fail in the second year, a remedial training placement will be arranged for a fixed period (typically 6 months), and if at the end of this time you still have not achieved the required competency level you will not receive a Foundation Achievement of Competency Document (FACD); and so cannot apply for specialty/core/GP training.

The foundation school director is obliged to inform the medical school and postgraduate deans if a foundation doctor has not been signed off at the expected time.

Sources of further information

NHS Foundation Programme: http://www.foundationprogramme.nhs.uk

Modernising Medical Careers: http://www.mmc.nhs.uk

NHS foundation support: http://www.nhscareers.nhs.uk/foundationtraining

4

Core and specialty training

Key aims of this chapter

- Give an overview of the process of applying to core/specialty training
- Give guidance on how to apply and where to go for further information.

Introduction

It is worthwhile thinking about the specialty programme you want to apply to as a foundation doctor, as applications will need to be completed partway through your F2 training. If you really do not have any inclinations towards one specialty or another, then it's not a disaster and you don't need to panic. With Modernising Medical Careers (MMC), you can keep a relatively broad base to your training until relatively late in your career – typically ST3 level for most specialties. You will however need to decide which broad area in medicine you want to pursue, e.g. medicine, surgery or general practice.

Specialty training

In general, specialty training programmes can be either 'run-through' or 'uncoupled' (see Table 4.1), the exception being orthopaedics, where both uncoupled and run-though programmes are available, and this depends on the deanery.

Run-through specialty training programmes

Run-through training programmes offer seamless progression (provided you meet the required competencies) to the endpoint of training.

Table 4.1: An overview of specialties that offer run-through versus those that offer 'uncoupled' training

Specialties that offer run-through training	Specialties that offer uncoupled training
Obstetrics and gynaecology – application can also be made at ST2 and ST3	Anaesthesia
Ophthalmology – application can also be made at ST2 and ST3	Core medical training, with competitive entry to 28 medical specialties at ST3
Paediatrics and child health – application can also be made at ST2, ST3 and ST4	Core surgical training, with competitive entry to 9 surgical specialties at ST3
General practice	Emergency medicine (core training is for 3 years)
Public health medicine	Psychiatry (core training is for 3 years)
Trauma and Orthopaedic Surgery	Trauma and Orthopaedic Surgery
Neurosurgery – application can also be made at ST2 and ST3	
Histopathology	
Chemical pathology	
Medical microbiology/virology	
Clinical radiology (applicants can apply from foundation training or following completion of core training within another specialty)	

The specialty training (ST) years in these types of programme are termed ST1, ST2, ST3 etc.

In other specialties, training is 'uncoupled' and following core training (CT), which can be for either 2 or 3 years. There will be open competition to ST3 and ST4, respectively. Core training is a term that encompasses:

● Core medical training
● Acute care common stem
● Core surgical training
● Core psychiatric training.

Generally speaking all of these core training programmes, with the exception of psychiatry, are for a period of 2 years. In psychiatry, core training is for 3 years. Trainees in core training, like trainees at the equivalent level in specialties continuing with run-through training, are termed 'specialty registrars' (StRs). This distinguishes them from SpRs (specialist registrars) – those trainees taking up appointment in these specialties before the introduction of core specialty training.

It is important to remember that where training is uncoupled, competition into ST3 (4) posts will be high, as not only will you be in competition with ST2s, but you will also be in competition with doctors caught in between the old and new training systems, those who are currently in research or within fixed-term specialty training appointment (FTSTA) posts and others who may have taken a period out of medicine – so there will be far more applicants than posts available.

Career progression following core training

The Acute Care Common Stem (ACCS) has within it a number of themed specialty groups that are available in the first 2 years of the programme:

- Acute medicine – following this a further themed third year in emergency medicine needs to be undertaken in order to apply for an ST4 in emergency medicine
- Anaesthesia/critical care – following this, a third year in anaesthesia at CT2 level can be undertaken and this will allow competitive application for ST3 anaesthesia
- Emergency medicine.

Completion of an acute medicine-themed ACCS programme can open a number of doors for you – and will make you eligible for entry to training at ST3 into the medical specialties, and for entry at ST4 into emergency medicine, and ST3 into anaesthesia.

Following core surgical training, which is for 2 years, application can be made at ST3 into the following specialties:

- Cardiothoracic surgery
- General surgery
- ENT
- Paediatric surgery
- Plastic surgery
- Trauma and orthopaedics
- Urology
- Oral and maxillofacial surgery (OMFS).

After core training in psychiatry, which is for 3 years (CT1-3), application at ST4 can be made to:

- Child and adolescent psychiatry
- General adult psychiatry
- Old-age psychiatry
- Forensic psychiatry
- Psychotherapy.

Following core medical training, application to 28 themed medical specialties at ST3 is possible. These specialties include:

- Allergy
- Audiological medicine
- Cardiology
- Clinical genetics
- Clinical neurophysiology
- Clinical oncology
- Clinical pharmacology and therapeutics
- Dermatology
- Endocrinology and diabetes
- Gastroenterology
- Genitourinary medicine
- Geriatric medicine
- Haematology
- Immunology
- Infectious diseases
- Medical microbiology
- Medical oncology
- Medical ophthalmology
- Neurology
- Nuclear medicine
- Occupational medicine
- Palliative medicine
- Paediatric cardiology
- Rehabilitation medicine
- Renal medicine
- Respiratory medicine
- Rheumatology
- Sports medicine
- Tropical medicine.

Fixed-term specialty training appointments

FTSTAs are 1-year stand-alone appointments that exist in those specialties that have retained run-through training. They are posts that are recognised for training, and may be of benefit if you are looking for an additional year's experience, or if you perhaps need a further year's training in order to meet the eligibility criteria for higher specialty training posts. For example, if you have completed 2 years of core medical training and a third year is needed before you can apply for a particular paediatrics post. Notably, if you do take up an FTSTA post, the chances of you obtaining a run-through post at ST2 will be lower, since there will be very few of these posts available. In the future, FTSTAs will be absorbed into core training programmes and therefore will not exist.

Endpoint of training

Completion of core training allows you to compete for higher specialty training programmes within the formal career grade structure. It does not however automatically entitle or guarantee you a place on a further specialty training programme. Following successful completion of higher specialty training you will be awarded a CCT, Certificate confirming Eligibility to the Specialist Register (CESR) or Certificate confirming Eligibility to the GP Register (CEGPR), as appropriate, and this will qualify you for entry to the Specialist or GP Register, which is held by the GMC.

Applying for specialty training

Anyone who meets the person specification for entry into core/specialty/ GP training is eligible to apply for specialty training. The criterion outlined in the person specification is standardised and therefore the same across the country for any given specialty. Importantly, for entry at ST1 and CT1 you cannot have held a post for $\geq$18 months in the specialty to which you are applying by the time you take up that post.

Person specifications can be found for each medical specialty on training websites and are assessed for using both the application form and an interview process. The person specification will differ for each specialty, but each will have a similar framework. Each strand for selection is given an 'essential' or 'desirable' banding, and perhaps unsurprisingly the more 'desirable' criteria you possess the more likely it is you will be shortlisted. It is well worthwhile as an F1 or F2 to have a look at the person specification for the specialty you are interested in and work towards fulfilling as much of not only the essential, but also the desirable criteria as possible.

An overview of the person specification for core medical training (CT1) is given as an example below:

1. **Qualifications**
   - MBBS or equivalent (essential)
   - Postgraduate examinations, e.g. Membership of the Royal College of Physicians (MRCP) (essential).

2. **Eligibility to practice**
   - Eligible for full GMC registration at the time of appointment; in some cases a current license to practice is also required (essential)
   - Evidence of achieving foundation competencies in line with *Good Medical Practice* (essential).

3. **Eligibility to work in the UK (essential)**
   - In the case of overseas applicants, evidence of immigration status, together with a letter from the Home Office detailing your type of visa, will need to be provided and dated not after the closing date for applications for the post you are applying to.

4. **Fitness to practice**
   - Is up to date and fit to practice (essential).

5. **Language skills**
   - Possess adequate and demonstrable written and spoken skills in English (essential)
   - If your medical school training was not in English, you will need to provide evidence supporting your English language skills, e.g. valid English Language Testing System (IELTS 7.0) certificate.

6. **Health**
   - Meets professional health standards in line with *Good Medical Practice* (essential).

7. **Career progression**
   - Ability to provide appointment history (essential)
   - 12 months or less experience at senior house officer (SHO) level in given specialty by job start date, not including foundation modules (essential).

8. **Completion of the application form**
   - All sections of the application form completed fully (essential).

9. **Clinical skills**
   - Appropriate knowledge base and sound clinical judgement (essential).

10. **Academic/research skills**
    - Demonstrates an understanding of the importance of research and audit (essential)
    - Evidence of academic and research interest, participation in audit and teaching (desirable).

11. **Personal skills**
    - Vigilance and situational skills (essential)
    - Coping under pressure (essential)
    - Communication skills (essential)
    - Problem-solving and decision-making skills (essential)
    - Managing others and team involvement (essential)
    - Organisation and planning (essential)
    - Empathy and sympathy (essential).

12. **Probity**
    - Professional integrity (essential).

13. **Commitment to specialty**
    - Learning and development (essential)
    - Extracurricular activities/achievements relevant to specialty (desirable).

Sending off the application

Recruitment into specialty training programmes in the UK for most specialties is via a single online application through a central office for

One of the essential criteria for appointment to a specialty training programme is evidence of achievement of foundation or equivalent competences. If you have undertaken a foundation programme in the UK, at the end of your training you will be awarded a Certificate of Completion of Foundation training (FACD 5.2), and this needs to be made available to your employer on starting your post, if successful. FACDs can take time to process and you will therefore need to have completed all of your foundation assessments, at least 1 month ahead of the date of actual completion of your foundation programme to be able to process your FACD in time for your next post.

If you did not train in a UK foundation programme, you will need to submit alternative evidence of achieving the equivalent competencies, and you should contact your local deanery to clarify how this may be achieved.

Box 4.1 Evidence of achievement of foundation or equivalent competencies selection, so you will only need to submit one application form for any one specialty, ranking your deanery by order of preference. Importantly, you are not limited to or penalised if you apply to more than one specialty and you should consider doing so, especially if you think your application may be weak or if you are applying for a very competitive specialty. This is an approach that should be considered and adopted from the onset, rather than midway through the application process, as a panic measure, when you fail to be shortlisted for your first-choice specialty.

There are two channels or offices through which your application can be managed:

1. The Royal Colleges, and specialties currently recruiting in this manner are:
   - Obstetrics and gynaecology, through the Royal College of Obstetrics and Gynaecology for all levels
   - Paediatrics and Child Health, through the Royal College of Paediatrics and Child Health for all levels
   - Core Medical Training, through the Royal College of Physicians, for CT1 only
   - Psychiatry, through the Royal College of Psychiatry, for CT1 and CT4.

2. The deaneries, whereby a single deanery is charged as the 'lead' deanery and is responsible for running the application process for that particular specialty. Specialties recruiting through a lead deanery include:
   - Public Health, through the East Midlands Deanery, for ST1
   - Clinical Radiology, through the London Deanery for ST1
   - Histopathology, through the London Deanery for ST1
   - General Practice, through the National Recruitment Office, for ST1
   - Anaesthetics, through the West Midlands Deanery, for CT2 and ST3
   - Neurosurgery, through the Yorkshire and the Humber Deanery, for all levels.

Advertising of specialist training posts

Each recruiting office is responsible for advertising posts, providing information about the posts within a rotation (where available) and overseeing the recruitment process, i.e. receiving and shortlisting applications in accordance with nationally agreed standards, interviewing (as well as providing information regarding the shortlisting criteria and any scoring scheme used as well as the interview methodology), making job offers to successful candidates and handling any appeals/complaints.

The timetable for applications including both opening and closing dates, and shortlisting and interview dates should be available in advance on the recruiting office website. Posts are required to be advertised at least 2 weeks ahead, so you should keep your eyes open for these and aim to apply well ahead of the closure of the applications deadline. In addition, it is worthwhile contacting your referees well ahead of time to check they will be able to complete the structured references in good time.

Job vacancies may also be posted by individual deaneries on the NHS Jobs website or in Job Centre Plus as well as in publications such as BMJ Careers, though this is not a requirement. You should keep your eyes peeled for these vacancies. If you have any questions regarding the recruiting process, you should contact the email helpdesk services at the relevant deanery; they are obliged to respond to any applicant query within 48 hours. In some deaneries, a recruitment telephone helpline may also be available.

The first and main recruitment round for recruitment to CT1/ST1 specialty training programmes typically starts at the end of the year and will usually end by Easter of the following year; this process is co-ordinated nationally. If you do not secure a post in round 1 of applications, you do have another shot, as round 2 of recruitment will follow shortly after and can even overlap round 1 of recruitment; however, no round 2 job offers will be made until the first round has been completed fully. The second round of recruitment will include unfilled posts from round 1, as well as previously unadvertised CT2/ST2, CT3 and ST3 posts. Importantly, if you have accepted a post in round 1 and for whatever reason re-apply in round 2 and accept the second post; you will need to give or work the required period of notice before taking up the second post.

Selection to specialty programmes

All shortlisted candidates will be interviewed by their recruiting office by representatives of the different training programmes throughout the UK and those candidates selected at interview will be offered the available posts. The top-ranked candidate at interview will almost certainly get their first-choice post, the second-ranked will then be given their choice of post and so forth down the ranks.

Deciding on the specialty for you – things to consider

Everyone's idea of the perfect job is different and no one medical specialty will suit all. Before applying for a specialty programme you need to take a hard look at the factors that attract you to a specialty as well as its downsides. If you haven't decided on a specialty yet, then it's worthwhile listing the factors that motivate you as well as your attributes and how they may best be accommodated by the specialties available. A question worth asking yourself is: 'Where do you see yourself in 10 years' time?'

A number of factors are likely to influence which specialty you apply to and the deanery to which you apply:

- Your personality (including your values, aspirations, strengths and weaknesses)
- The way healthcare is changing in terms of its delivery
- Your personal life, e.g. children, lifestyle expectations
- Levels of competition for a specialty or region
- Geography
- The strength of your application.

Competition

You should definitely take into account the competition for posts into account when applying for specialty training. Some specialties such as clinical radiology, core surgical training and public health, amongst others, are extremely popular and unless you have a very strong application, it is worth being flexible about your choice of specialty and having a back-up plan in place. In addition, the number of posts available in certain specialties is likely to change in the future, largely in response to changes in the way healthcare will be delivered. It is predicted that approximately half of the training posts in the future will be in general practice, and the number of posts in surgical specialties will be reduced.

Location

The level of competition for a specialty programme will also be determined by deanery applied to, and if you are not bound by geography, it is well worthwhile ranking less popular deaneries higher for any given specialty; this approach is especially encouraged if your application is weak.

It is well worth discussing your application with your educational/clinical supervisor or a mentor, to gauge the strength of your application, and the likelihood of you being shortlisted for a given specialty and/or region.

Other people or places you could seek careers advice from include:

- Senior colleagues, e.g. consultants
- Deanery career advisor or support team
- Postgraduate dean
- Your foundation programme director
- Your Trust's director of medical education or careers lead
- Royal College tutors
- Web resources: www.medicalcareers.nhs.uk
- Careers days
- The British Medical Association's Doctors for Doctors Unit, which is useful for doctors in distress or difficulty or under pressure.

Whatever specialty or specialties you apply to, you need to do your homework beforehand, i.e. look at the person specifications, ensure your portfolio is up-to-date, and research the post and whether you would be suited to it; this may involve speaking to as many people as possible within that specialty or organising a 'taster' period. There are no two ways about it, the application process is stressful, however you are not alone and there are plenty of other people who are in exactly the same position. The key is to try and be as flexible as possible and have a back-up plan in place should things not go quite as planned.

Options for careers in academic medicine

If you were on the AFP, you may very well wish to carry on your interest in research and there are a number of avenues through which you can pursue this, for example:

- Clinical lectureships – these allow you to undertake an academic training programme alongside your clinical training programme. Typically your time will be split 80/20 between clinical work and research activity, and there is some flexibility regarding the proportions of time spent within each (as long as the time spent in clinical training does not fall below 50%).
- University or CSO Fellowships – these are similar to clinical lectureships in England and Northern Ireland and allow you to perform postdoctoral research work whilst in clinical training. These may lead to Scottish Senior Clinical Fellowships or Clinician Scientist Fellowship appointments.
- A number of local variations of academic programmes also exist, for example, Edinburgh University offers doctors in specialty training an

Table 4.2: Competition for specialty training positions (taken from www.mmc.co.uk). Posts, applications and shortlisting information by specialty for entry level ST1 posts

Specialty	Theme	Number of posts	Applications		Shortlistings		Applications per post		Shortlistings per post		% of applications shortlisted	
			All	1st choices	All	1st choices	All	1st choices	All	1st choices	All	1st choices
Acute Care Common Stem (ACCS)	Acute medicine	78	722	119	252	46	9.3	1.5	3.2	0.6	35%	39%
Acute Care Common Stem (ACCS)	Anaesthesia	124	678	167	324	96	5.5	1.3	2.6	0.8	48%	57%
Acute Care Common Stem (ACCS)	Emergency medicine	248	2094	481	653	165	8.4	1.9	2.6	0.7	31%	34%
Acute Care Common Stem (ACCS)	Intensive care medicine	8	29	11	6	4	3.6	1.4	0.8	0.5	21%	36%
Anaesthesia		525	2538	637	1184	357	4.8	1.2	2.3	0.7	47%	56%
Chemical pathology		11	97	20	34	10	8.8	1.8	3.1	0.9	35%	50%
Clinical radiology		184	3325	848	591	163	18.1	4.6	3.2	0.9	18%	19%
Core medical training		1338	7781	1934	2829	807	5.8	1.4	2.1	0.6	36%	42%
General practice		2515	15406	4241	4982	3118	6.1	1.7	2.0	1.2	32%	74%
Histopathology		87	757	296	210	109	8.7	3.4	2.4	1.3	28%	37%
Medical microbiology & virology			1	1							0%	0%

Specialty	Subspecialty											
Medical microbiology & virology	Med micro	23	415	93	89	22	18.0	4.0	3.9	1.0	21%	24%
Medical microbiology & virology	Virology	3	16	7	9	3	5.3	2.3	3.0	1.0	56%	43%
Neurosurgery		35	262	76	100	36	7.5	2.2	2.9	1.0	38%	47%
Obstetrics & gynaecology		289	2023	514	812	219	7.0	1.8	2.8	0.8	40%	43%
Ophthalmology		110	906	260	243	84	8.2	2.4	2.2	0.8	27%	32%
Oral & maxillofacial surgery (OMFS)		25	219	59	103	29	8.8	2.4	4.1	1.2	47%	49%
Paediatrics		458	2047	511	927	253	4.5	1.1	2.0	0.6	45%	50%
Psychiatry		594	3040	713	1139	311	5.1	1.2	1.9	0.5	37%	44%
Public health		69	1242	370	193	72	18.0	5.4	2.8	1.0	16%	19%
Surgery in general	Cardiothoracic surgery	9	19	7	10	4	2.1	0.8	1.1	0.4	53%	57%
Surgery in general	General surgery	267	1804	432	497	135	6.8	1.6	1.9	0.5	28%	31%
Surgery in general	Generic	218	1404	487	470	179	6.4	2.2	2.2	0.8	33%	37%
Surgery in general	Otolaryngology (ENT)	68	300	83	130	41	4.4	1.2	1.9	0.6	43%	49%
Surgery in general	Paediatric surgery	15	78	22	47	11	5.2	1.5	3.1	0.7	60%	50%
Surgery in general	Plastic	44	357	98	105	28	8.1	2.2	2.4	0.6	29%	29%

academic run-through programme, and similar run-through academic schemes also exist in Wales. These types of schemes can be for a period of up to 8 years and include a 3-year PhD programme.

Frequently asked questions

Can I train flexibly?

The option to train flexibility does exist, however, in order to train flexibly you will need to prove that you could not practically train full time. You should discuss this option with your deanery following your appointment to a specialty programme.

Can non-UK/EAA applicants apply for specialty training?

Non-UK/EEA applicants can only apply for specialty training during round 2 of the recruitment process. In order to apply, like UK/EEA applicants you will need to meet the person specifications for the post you are applying to and this includes fulfilling UK immigration rules.

Can I defer the start of core training or take time out of programme?

You can only defer the start of core training if there are mitigating circumstances, e.g. ill health or maternity leave. If you are considering this, you should discuss it with your postgraduate dean at the earliest opportunity. Notably, out-of-programme (OOP) experiences will not usually be approved until a trainee has been within a training programme for at least 1 year, except in exceptional cases.

Can I transfer between deaneries?

Inter-deanery transfers are possible, however trainees usually should have been in post for a minimum of 1 year, unless there are exceptional circumstances. All transfers need to be discussed and approved by your postgraduate deans.

Sources of further information

NHS Foundation Programme: http://www.foundationprogramme.nhs.uk
Modernising Medical Careers: http://www.mmc.nhs.uk

NHS foundation support: http://www.nhscareers.nhs.uk/foundationtraining

GP Training: http://gprecruitment.org.uk

Recruitment to medical specialty training in Scotland: http://www.mmc.scot.nhs.uk

Recruitment to medical specialty training in Wales: http://www.mmcwales.org

Recruitment to medical specialty training in Northern Ireland: http://www.nimdta.gov.uk

Academic posts: http://www.nihrtcc.nhs.uk

5

Specialty training application forms

Key aims of this chapter

- Describe the processes involved with applying for clinical jobs
- Detail examples of general questions with real-life answers
- Detail examples of scenario-based questions with real-life answers.

Introduction

Application forms for training positions are now widespread within the UK. For certain non-training positions, such as 6-month Clinical Fellow posts, the requirement may simply be a covering letter with CV. However, the vast majority of positions require a detailed form to be filled in as part of the application process. This generic system may actually make it harder for individual applicants to stand out. In addition, although some of the questions seem straightforward, it is vital to understand what the shortlisting committee are looking for as this is not always apparent at first glance.

Application process

Once positions are advertised, the application forms are almost always available on the Internet. It can be difficult to find the exact locations of forms and it is important to check individual deanery sites for specific web locations and dates of release. Forms should be downloaded and filled in on screen. The maximum word count should be adhered to (the sections of the forms are usually closed to stop an excess of words) and in most cases the word limit should be reached. The forms are then sent off either by post or email (or sometimes both).

Some websites may also give a person specification, detailing ideal attributes that they are seeking in trainees. These may not necessarily be the same for hospital specialties and general practice, and should be borne in mind when completing the application form. For example, those interested in general practice can download a (Department of Health approved) person specification, and other useful information from the National Office for GP recruitment. This becomes especially useful if you are unsure as to what to write in a question asking what 'qualities' you will bring to a specialty, or what makes you think you will be a good doctor in your chosen specialty as you can then tailor your answer to the person specification.

The exact application form will vary between deaneries and specialties but in reality many are similar in the style of questions asked. There are often two main sections. Firstly, there are standardised questions asking for generic information. These are used simply for administrative purposes. Any information regarding ethnicity, disability and sexual orientation may be asked for on a specific part of the form but this will not be seen by the shortlisting committee and indeed there is often a box marked 'not disclosed' if you do not wish to answer such information.

The standard generic questions at the beginning of an application form typically include questions regarding personal details such as your name, telephone number and address, your GMC registration number, your immigration status and your language skills. For GP applications, a full UK driving licence is also required.

There will also be a fitness to practice section where you have to make it clear that you are free to practice with no (or some limited) restrictions set by the GMC. You will additionally have to detail whether or not you have any criminal convictions. The section on core competencies may be taken from your log book and will show that you have achieved the necessary skills to apply for the post. It is important to list your previous jobs in chronological order with details of the senior doctors you have worked for. If there is space, you should list the key clinical and managerial responsibilities of each post. The references section is usually at the end of the application form and you should contact your referees prior to the application process to inform them that they may be contacted.

The second part of the form will deal with two types of questions. Firstly, there are general questions that can be applicable to almost any field. These include sections on core competencies, audit and academic achievements. The questions will differ according to type of position, e.g. for an Academic Training Fellowship the bulk of questions may revolve around research experience but for a surgical specialty the questions may concern practical skills.

The second set of questions (which is not always encountered) regards scenario-based questions. These allow the applicant to give details of specific instances to help the shortlisting committee decide whom to invite for interview.

Shortlisting scores vary between deaneries but in general each question on the form is marked. The total scores are collated and the top percentage of applicants will be invited to interview. As many applicants fill in the questions in a similar way it is important to try to distinguish yourself from the crowd. Often, these may be with specific exam qualifications, research or with experience in a particular field. However, the actual method of answering the questions can greatly improve your chances of getting to interview.

General questions

All of the questions shown below are taken from current application forms for medical training jobs in the UK. For each question shown, there is an

There are a number of companies that specialise in drafting answers for application forms. These companies may either speak to applicants to help prepare answers or write the entire application forms from scratch based on a few answers supplied by candidates. However, aside from the costs involved, it is often better to complete the form yourself based on your own CV and actual experiences. In general it should be remembered that:

- There are no key words that the shortlisting committee are looking for; rather they are looking for the general approach to a question
- They will be considering whether the applicant has truly understood the question
- They will try to determine whether the answer is honest and representative of the applicant's experience
- Many deaneries use plagiarism software so answers copied verbatim are likely to be discovered and given a score of zero, or may even result in your application form being rejected outright or even possible referral to the GMC for misconduct.

Box 5.1 Companies that specialise in filling in application forms and tips to keep in mind insight into what the shortlisting committee are looking for as well as a real-life example (taken from recent application forms) of an answer that has the potential to score top marks in the shortlisting process.

Question

What clinical knowledge and experience do you have that is particular to this post (ST1 in core medicine)? (*250 words*)

This question aims to ensure that you have enough clinical experience for the post. It is important to stress if you have worked in the same specialty at a junior level and also detail any practical procedures that you may be competent with. It is also vital not to over emphasise your skills as you may be seen as arrogant and overconfident. Whatever post you apply for, you will be learning in that new job. In order to achieve top marks for this question you need to stress where you have areas that are particularly deficient and what you would do to remedy this.

Answer

By August 2011 I will have completed 24 months of foundation training, including acute medicine, neurology, endocrinology, general practice and emergency medicine at St Dean's Hospital (a level 1 trauma centre). When on-call, I am happy to be first to see patients, perform appropriate investigations and instigate management. I enjoy seeing admissions that have challenging diagnoses and often review patients seen by FY1 doctors and medical students before they present to the SpR.

As part of my neurology FY2 I was the specialist on-call overnight (1 in 10 rota) with the on-call consultant as my next port of advice.

I play an active role in cardiac arrests and aim to lead if I am the senior doctor first on site until the medical registrar or anaesthetist arrives. I am becoming more confident at being the first person to review sick medical patients on the wards and start emergency management. However, I realise my own limitations with such patients and will always immediately call for senior help if I am unsure of what to do.

I have attended a series of postgraduate courses including Intermediate Life Support, Alert and Emergency Simulation. I have not yet completed an ALS course but in order to ensure that I am ready for my core medical training I have booked myself onto a course later this year. I am fully independent in a number of procedures including lumbar punctures, joint aspiration, arterial blood gases and pleural taps. I strongly feel that by August I will be ready to start core medical training.

Question

Please describe your level of clinical audit including details of your own involvement (*175 words*)

Most applicants will have been involved in audit either at medical school or as a junior doctor and so it is important to stand out from the crowd. If you initiated the audit then you should detail your reasoning for investigating the problem. You should discuss any difficulties associated with the audit and then explain how it was presented and who this was to. If there have been any changes then write about who made these changes and how they impacted on the clinical problem. If there are plans for a re-audit then this should also be detailed.

The shortlisting committee is not looking for a candidate who has created the most elaborate audit that has had wide-reaching implications. Such statements would be seen as overambitious. Instead, they are looking for real evidence of a thought process behind the creation of an audit to show them that as a member of a clinical team you could employ the same rational thinking and problem solving to patient care.

Answer

As an ST1 trainee in Derby I became concerned about the time taken for suspected heart attack patients to have inpatient exercise treadmill tests. I noticed that those given outpatient appointments were having fast investigations but for some reason those that were admitted to hospital had to wait for quite long periods of time. Often this was because they had other medical problems that the clinical teams felt needed sorting out and so the investigation was delayed.

I devised and carried out an audit reviewing 46 patients over 6 months, comparing times to National Institute for Clinical Excellence (NICE) guidelines. I presented the data to a meeting that I called for the Acute Medicine, Cardiology and Cardiac Testing departments.

I discussed recommendations to reduce this time, including a more detailed chest pain proforma and exercise tests that could take place towards the end of the day and could be reported by cardiologists in the morning. Some of my suggestions were implemented and my audit will be repeated this year.

Question

Please state whether you have made any oral or poster presentations and whether presented at regional, national or international meetings and give full titles (*350 words*)

This question is aimed to allow candidates who worked hard outside of their normal duties to show this to the shortlisting panel. Presentations at large meetings will be scored highly but even those that have been in your own hospital or medical school will be awarded points. It is important to emphasise the role that you took in the presentation and also why you were at the meeting. This will give the panel an insight into your commitment to the specialty.

Answer

1. *I delivered an oral presentation on 'Patient Satisfaction on the Wards' to the Yorkshire Regional Meeting of Gastroenterologists (comprising clinicians from five different hospitals) in December 2010. This was because I had carried out an audit into patient satisfaction in conjunction with my consultant, who suggested it to me during my ST1 job. The results (as well as suggestions for improving patient satisfaction) were presented to an audience of over 50 members of multidisciplinary staff from the hospitals. I will present the same audit results to the British Gastroenterology meeting in Spring 2011.*

2. *I presented a seminar on 'The use of non-invasive ventilation in patients with dementia' to a joint meeting of the Neurology, Respiratory and ICU departments at Manchester's Royal Infirmary in May 2010. I reviewed current NICE recommendations, evidence-based guidelines as well some of the latest high-impact publications and discussed areas of our care that needed improvement. This seminar was part of a day of teaching organised by the ICU department and I was asked to deliver it due to my interest in the non-invasive ventilation that had been used on one our patients whilst I was on the stroke team.*

3. *I helped create some hospital guidelines for heparin prophylaxis whilst I was an FY2 trainee in Leeds and I presented these guidelines to the hospital's monthly surgical meeting of morbidity and mortality. I had realised that some patients were being prescribed heparin on a haphazard basis. I carried out an audit looking into this and collected data prescriptions, comparing them to current NICE guidelines. One of my main findings was that some urology patients commencing*

inpatient therapy had no prophylaxis as they were being admitted on a short-stay ward where the drug charts were written before being transferred across to the main surgical ward. I gave an oral presentation of this to the meeting and the urology team have now changed the admissions process to ensure that all appropriate patients are given thromboprophylaxis.

Question

Give details of any of your academic achievements (*150 words*)

Again, the level of achievement here is what stands out with the more prestigious awards carrying higher marks. However, it is important to detail all awards that you have gained, even if you feel they may not be significant for this particular post. They should be listed by date with the title of the award and some idea as to how important it was.

Answer

1. Basic Sciences Prize for 1st MB exams awarded by University College London (May 2000). This award is given to only one candidate per year and is presented for the highest combined scores in all medical school first-year examinations.
2. General Practice Award as part of undergraduate Professional Development Spine for Essay on Elderly Care in the Community (June 2004). This award is given to the top three essays in general practice each year.
3. Overall prize in undergraduate epidemiology for essay and presentation entitled Health After a Natural Disaster awarded by University College London (June 2005). This award was for the best essay of the year in the epidemiology undergraduate course at the University.

Question

Have you been involved in teaching and how did you find the experience? (*250 words*)

Many applicants at the ST stage and above will have been involved with teaching. This may range from informal bedside teaching to medical students attached to a hospital firm to teaching on a postgraduate course for specialist exams. It is important to show that if you have been involved with teaching you have done so to a range of students across the disciplines of healthcare. In addition, even if not explicitly asked, you should detail the difficulties with teaching as well as what you may have learned yourself from the experience.

Answer

At Basildon general hospital I taught clinical skills to final-year medical students preparing for their OSCE exams. This teaching formed part of an official rota set up by University College London medical school in conjunction with the hospital. I was able to take four students at a time and give them bedside teaching on several occasions over a 3-month period. In addition, my FY2 job in a teaching hospital meant that students were able to observe me in outpatient clinics. When on-call for acute medicine I also try to teach basic practical procedures such as venesection and catheter insertion.

When I was an ST2 trainee in Liverpool I taught junior nurses from the local university that were attached to the Endocrine department. This was as part of the University's teaching schedule that I volunteered to teach on. I gave a series of seminars on diabetic foot care and antibiotic use and prepared some teaching notes that I handed onto the nurse-in-charge so that he could use them for the following years.

In general I have found teaching to be extremely rewarding. When teaching medical students and junior doctors I am sometimes confronted with questions that I do not know the answer to and whilst it is tempting to give a hazy answer I have found that it is often better to say that I am not sure but that I will find out and let them know. Whilst this can be difficult and time consuming it does help me improve my own knowledge.

Question

Provide evidence of your organisational skills with particular emphasis to show that you can complete or finish a task (*150 words*)

This is an opportunity for you to show that you can work within a medical team and organise the care of patients. This may be as a junior doctor organising the ward round and the list of jobs for different patients or it may be as a senior clinician managing the on-call rota within a specialty. In all regards the panel want to see that you have strong evidence of organisational skills. The example given does not necessarily have to be from within medicine but it must show how you *are able to tackle a major problem and organise people or resources to best manage the situation. It is also important to relate those skills learnt to the job you are applying for.*

As a medical student in Edinburgh I was appointed as the Chief Executive Officer for a 2-year term within the main charitable body at the University. My responsibilities included interviewing for key members of staff, dealing with accounts and organising fundraising events. I regularly headed up committee meetings and had a key management role, which meant I spent time on the main University's academic panel.

This experience has meant that I am better able to work as an ST3 in radiology. The leadership skills that I had to learn for the charity means that I will be better able to look after my patients and once I become a consultant I will be better able to manage the resources within my department.

Question

Is there any other professional experience that you would like to be taken into consideration (e.g. relevant courses attended)? (*200 words*)

It is important to list all courses and qualifications here that have not been listed elsewhere. The fixed nature of many application forms means that there is often no space to put this information. In the most extreme cases there is even no space for Royal College postgraduate exams so it is vital that these are listed first as they are the most important qualification in the shortlisting process. All others should be listed chronologically and any that are not standard should be explained in little detail.

I have passed the first two parts of the MRCP exams at the first attempt (part 1 in July 2010 and part 2 in December 2010). I am planning on sitting the final part (part 2 clinical examination [PACES]) in July 2011, by which time I feel I will have gained the clinical experience necessary to sit the exam. My other relevant qualifications are as follows:

- *Basic Life Support Training (July 2009)*
- *Advanced Life Support Training (December 2009)*

- Direct Response Workshop for ST Training (January 2010). This course was designed to allow new ST trainees to become competent in recognising sick patients and taught me how to initiate emergency immediate treatment
- Management course at London School of Business (February 2010). This is an online course that required 30 hours of work to complete and gave me an insight into management with a strong emphasis on leadership of teams of differing abilities. Although the course is designed for those in a business environment, I took it as I felt that it would help me once I become a consultant and have to manage a multidisciplinary team.

Question

Please enter evidence below of your publications [e.g. articles in magazines, journals with full citation, book chapter]. You MUST state clearly if the publication is an abstract, even if it is published in or as a supplement to, a peer-reviewed journal (*150 words*)

As with any question about academic awards, the quality of publications is what matters here. Obviously a first-author scientific paper in a prestigious journal would score highly but many doctors applying for junior positions will not have achieved this. It is important to detail all your publications and also explain your role in them as this may help score points. It is vital that you are completely honest as you may be asked to bring copies to an interview and any major twisting of the truth will be frowned upon.

Answer

I have written a number of articles both in medical school and as a junior doctor. These include:

1. *Simvastatin is shown to reduce mortality in wild-type mice with hypertension and inherent genetic cardiovascular morbidity. Elders J, Shah P, Michaels F, Smith R and Gurj P. BMJ 2008 Jan 27;353:b5634. This was a publication from my intercalated BSc degree in the pharmaceutical research group at the University of Manchester. My laboratory work on mice endothelium was included in the paper and I was given a middle authorship.*
2. *Medical management of asthma in the 21st century. Michaels F and Gray J. Book chapter in Medical Student Review Series. I co-authored this book chapter with my respiratory consultant whilst an ST2 at Manchester.*

3. *Review of patient compliance with anti-TNF alpha drugs. James G, Michaels F and Sandu J. Biosci Trends. 2010 Dec;7(6):210–19.I co-authored this review of patient compliance with my rheumatology professor and a final year SpR whilst I was in my first foundation year at Manchester.*

Question

How will this training programme and your previous training and experience help you meet your career objectives? What are your reasons for applying to this training programme? (*150 words*)

The shortlisting panel will want to know why you are applying for this particular job and how that makes you different from all the other applicants. This is your chance to show real enthusiasm for the specialty or deanery. As well as your reasons for applying you need to show that your experience in terms of junior jobs, practical procedures and patient interactions make you well suited for the post.

Answer

This training programme will allow me to initiate and carry out my own research projects leading towards my goal of becoming an academic vascular surgeon. I have published a number of research articles in the field including molecular work into arterial wall angiogenesis as part of my BSc project and epidemiological work looking into rates of stroke in the UK. These have been in peer-reviewed journals and in addition, I have presented at a number of national conferences.

The training programme will build on previous work from my ST1 and 2 posts in general surgery in London. I am now competent in a number of basic procedures (as evidenced by my log book) and have operated as a primary assistant to my consultant on a number of operations including endovenous ablation surgery and emergency aneurysm repair. I feel that acceptance on this training programme will help me to further my goals of becoming an academic vascular surgeon.

My long-term career goal is to work part time in clinical surgery and part time in laboratory research. To do this I would like to register for a higher degree such as an MD during my time as a specialist trainee and pursue this full time for 2 or 3 years before returning to finish my training.

Question

How can you demonstrate that you are committed to this specialty and why have you chosen it? (*250 words*)

This is a slight but important variation to the previous question. As well as showing why you are interested in working in the field you have to show an understanding of the difficulties involved in order to gain top marks. This will tell the shortlisting panel that you have really thought about a career in their area and weighed up both the pros and cons before making your decision.

Answer

After completing jobs in neurology, cardiology and respiratory medicine during my foundation years, I am convinced that I want to train in acute medicine. I really enjoy the daily challenges of dealing with extremely unwell patients and being able to stabilise them as soon as they come into hospital and then liaise with other specialist teams such as the Intensive Care department.

My FY2 year ends with 4 months in emergency medicine at the Barnet General Hospital in London. I chose this busy district general hospital as part of my foundation years as I am sure to learn a great deal that will be invaluable to me in my future career. I have taken my MRCP part 1 in January (my earliest available opportunity) and if successful will take the part 2 in July.

I have spoken to a number of consultants and other senior doctors in acute medicine, anaesthetics, intensive care and emergency medicine. I realise that there are many difficulties to life as an acute medicine physician including the long hours and a demanding workload, as well as the political problems that I am likely to face in the future of the NHS. However, taking all these into account, I am excited to meet such challenges and am sure that by August I will be ready to enter specialist training.

Question

Give brief details of all research projects and/or relevant research experience that you have undertaken or are undertaking, including methods used. Indicate your level of involvement and your exact role in the research team. (*175 words*)

As with a question on publications the more prestigious research posts will score higher marks. This is particularly relevant when applying for academic positions but similar questions (with lower expectations) may be found on general training application forms as well. It is important that your exact role is explained and not overemphasised as this may be probed in detail during an interview.

Answer

As part of my intercalated BSc degree I have published a proof of principle study examining T-cell responses to novel antigens in tuberculosis. This was laboratory work that I carried out over a 3-month period and I contributed to one figure in the paper (which was published in the Journal of Immunology). As an FY2 trainee in Bristol I participated in a clinical study examining the effect of statins on patients with diabetes and stroke. This was part of a large clinical trial that was published in the Journal of Molecular Biology. Although I was not listed as a prinicpal author, I was thanked by name in the manuscript for helping to recruit patients for the study.

I completed two audits during my FY2 and ST1 jobs. These were on postoperative complications of aortic abdominal aneurysm repair and the use of nasogastric (NG) feeding in patients with stroke. The second audit was presented at a regional meeting and I am in the process of writing it up for submission.

Question

What do you see are the advantages and disadvantages of a career in general practice? (*200 words*)

This question is not necessarily seeking the answer you might get from a careers guide. It is an opportunity to demonstrate what you have learned from student, elective and/or FY2 placements in general practice, as well as your insight from reading and networking. It should be as much about you as the job.

Answer

Advantages: As a medical student I enjoyed general practice attachments, particularly the variety of clinical problems and the challenge of coming to a diagnosis without immediate access to laboratory tests and radiological imaging. It was also a privilege to see the patients in context of their life.

The GPs I was placed with had a diverse array of special interests: one did minor surgery 1 afternoon a week, another ran a child health surveillance clinic. The GPs were also able to build knowledge of their patients and the local area. The ability to follow-up patients quickly and have booked appointments with some control over the workload on a given day is also appealing.

Disadvantages*: I can imagine that it can be isolating and there is often little opportunity between consultations to seek advice. GPs also manage a lot of uncertainty and there has been adverse publicity about missed diagnoses. In reading the BMJ, BMA News, and copies of GP Update, it is apparent that there is a widespread perception that it is becoming more difficult to obtain GP partnerships than it used to be, and a large number of newly qualified GPs opt to do salaried jobs or work as locums. I appreciate this may also be a positive choice, and allow a GP to pursue other interests.*

Question

How did you decide to pursue a career as GP? (*175 words*)

This question not only asks why you would like to be a GP, but allows you to provide some evidence of insight into the specialty. In short it provides an opportunity to relate your aims back to your experiences. A list of experience by itself may not be enough here.

Answer

As an undergraduate, I enjoyed my general practice placements. Some of my more inspiring undergraduate teachers have been GPs. They and others have given me a sense of the clinical variety and complexity that a career in general practice offers. As an undergraduate, I completed an intercalated BSc in Medical Ethics at King's College London. As my dissertation for the course I studied the ethical relevance of the differences in the doctor–patient relationship in hospital medicine compared to general practice – the key differences being the unfiltered nature of problems and the possibility for a longer interaction over many consultations over time in general practice.

As an FY2 doctor in general practice, I had the further opportunity to experience life as a GP, and with appropriate supervision to do home visits, plan management of chronic illness and deal with psycho–social problems in the community. I found these experiences intellectually stimulating and emotionally rewarding, such that I now aim to pursue a career as a GP.

Question

What two key qualities will you bring to a career as a GP?
(*300 words*)

Though there are no 'key words' and plagiarism may result in a application being rejected outright or worse, this question allows you to compare yourself to the qualities manifest in the person specification. If this is a real stretch of the imagination you should think twice about applying!

Consider what experiences you have had and how they relate to the desirable qualities. The person specification may be obtained from the GP recruitment website.

Answer

In my foundation year placements I enjoyed the opportunity to manage my work and at times was given the opportunity to lead the ward round and attend multidisciplinary meetings on behalf of the team. I was able to come up with management plans and checked these with a senior doctor. At the same time as allowing me to grow in confidence, these years have also re-emphasised the boundaries to my competence. I feel this awareness of limits to competence is also a valuable quality in a clinical environment that may sometimes appear isolated from the 'back up' of secondary medicine.

As an FY2 doctor I was elected as mess president. At the time the mess had few subscribers and was largely deserted. While president I instituted regular events with sponsorship, found out what members wanted and consequently obtained subscriptions. Whilst the mess had traditionally been a 'FY1-only' environment, I also encouraged FY2 and ST trainees to participate. This had an additional benefit of better working relationships between juniors of different levels on the wards. Where colleagues had an idea for a good event I allowed them to take a lead and provided whatever support was needed.

I also became involved in the local BMA Junior Doctors' Committee as the hospital representative, and was able to connect junior doctors who were having problems with the appropriate support. I feel that a good leader is able to delegate, and to be able to deal with and respond to the concerns of all members of the team. I imagine that this must have a special value in a general practice environment.

Question

Please say why you want an Academic Clinical Fellowship, indicating your medium and long-term career goals in relation to an academic career in this specialty. (*200 words*)

This question is specific to academic posts and must be answered cautiously. The shortlisting panel will expect all candidates to have shown an interest in research both as a medical student and as a junior doctor. You need to be extremely enthusiastic about pursuing a career both in research and in the particular specialty in question.

Answer

As a medical student in Aberdeen I was inspired by an academic consultant in psychiatry. She lectured at the University and was able to combine a clinical post with managing a research team and in addition have time for a family. I am interested in a career in academic psychiatry. If I am successful in applying for an academic training post I intend to immediately plan a research proposal to achieve funding towards a PhD. This will be in the area of child and adolescent psychiatry, in which I am most interested.

Once I have completed a period of research I would like to continue my clinical training whilst still pursuing a research career; this would be in the form of a clinical lectureship at a teaching hospital attached to a University. I would like to finally be appointed as an honorary consultant with a mix of both research and teaching in addition to my clinical work.

I know that Leeds has a world-renowned academic unit specialising in child and adolescent psychiatry and this is why I have applied to this post. I know that if I am appointed I will work to make sure I achieve the most that I can from the training scheme.

Question

Is there any further information that you would like to present to support your application? (*200 words*)

This is your opportunity to provide any information that you think is relevant but that you have not been able to slot into another section. It can be used to talk about extra-curricular activities, passions outside of medicine and interesting details from your career so far. It is also the chance to show your passion for the position in question. This is vital as

*this question is often the final one in an application form and so the final
thing a shortlisting panel will read before they make a decision about you.*

Answer

*My main passion outside of medicine and my family life is music. I
have attained grade 8 at piano and still take weekly lessons to improve
my technique. My passion for the works of Rachmaninov and other
contemporary composers has helped me deal with a career that is
sometimes busy and stressful.*

*I have also been involved with a charity to help orphans in Sri Lanka for
more than 5 years. As treasurer to the organisation my role has been to
raise funds, organise events and make sure that the accounts are up to
date. I have used my knowledge of technology to set up social networking
groups on sites like Facebook and Twitter and this has enabled me to
attract a new generation of donors to the charity.*

*I am taking my Member of the Royal College of Surgeons (MRCS)
examinations at the earliest possible opportunity and have passed the
first two parts at the first attempt. I am due to sit the final exam in June.
I feel that by August I will have achieved the necessary clinical skills and
theoretical knowledge to enter specialist training in surgery.*

Scenario-based questions

Question

**Give a recent example of when you have had to use your
communication and interpersonal skills (*250 words*)**

*This can be an example from outside medicine but whatever you write
about it must clearly explain a particular issue or problem and how your
own skills were used to solve it. In addition, you should explain how
you had learnt these skills. You should end by showing that although
the problem may have been solved, you had learnt something from the
situation and in the future you would be even more adept at managing
the situation.*

Answer

*As an ST1 in orthopaedic surgery I learnt to communicate with some
elderly patients who may have been healthy before having a fall and*

developing a fracture. One man was a successful businessman who had postoperatively developed a large myocardial infarction. Although he had slowly recovered from this he had become very depressed. I made it a point to speak to him and his family for a short period of time at the end of every day to talk through his progress.

I also arranged meetings between the surgical team and his family so that we could explain how things were evolving. Although I was a junior member of the team I was perhaps one of the most visible as I was on the wards every day and this was something that I took advantage of.

The patient needed a lot of hip and cardiac rehabilitation and he gradually began to improve with the input from our team. I feel that my daily encouragement played a part in this improvement. I learnt from this experience that as well as good communication with an unwell patient, it is vital to discuss any progress with family members. Once the doctors and nurses have left the bedside it is the family who are often responsible for ongoing encouragement and support. Once I become a senior doctor I will ensure that all members of my team speak to our patients' families whenever feasible.

Question

Give a recent example of when you have had to use your initiative (*200 words*)

Initiative is a quality that is highly sought after in medicine. Your answer must show that you possess the necessary qualities to find novel solutions to problems and exhibit leadership skills. The shortlisting panel will need to see this explained clearly. The example must be a personal one and it is useful to show something that has resulted in a real benefit for a patient or a system or practice.

Answer

As FY1 trainees in general surgery we were asked to cross-cover for the orthopaedic FY2 doctors when they were on annual leave or nights. I began to feel that this situation posed real clinical risk as patients from both teams were being less well managed.

I noticed that there were a number of orthopaedic Clinical Fellows who did not do on-calls and who were scheduled to do both surgery and clinics each day. I put forward a suggestion that the Clinical Fellows would cover for their own FY2 trainees. This would result in them missing one clinic a week and the orthopaedic consultants were unhappy with this.

As part of the joint surgery mortality and morbidity meeting I co-presented a case series of three patients with my SpR. These were instances of surgical or orthopaedic patients who had been given substandard care due to the cross-cover system. The orthopaedic consultants agreed and have subsequently changed the rota. This has resulted in better standards of care for both sets of surgical patients.

Question

Give a recent example of when you have had to deal with a difficult patient and/or family and what did you learn from this? (*250 words*)

This question is one that is also typically asked at interview. All applicants will have encountered such patients and the shortlisting panel are looking for evidence that you have dealt with the problem professionally and allowed the patient or family member to see their complaint through to a conclusion. They will also want to see that you have learnt from any mistakes you or others may have made during the process.

Answer

As an ST1 trainee in paediatrics we treated a young girl with meningitis. She had been assessed by the Emergency department but they had not involved the paediatricians until a few hours into her treatment. She was extremely unwell and although she made a good recovery her parents wanted to make a complaint about the care given to her in the Emergency Medicine department and asked for my advice.

As a junior member of the team I did not want to influence their thoughts so I explained that I would speak to my consultant and ask her to sit down with the parents. I did however explain that although we were involved after a few hours, their daughter had been given the highest possible care by the emergency team. I think it is important that if serious complaints are going to be made you should involve the most senior member of the team and not unduly influence the patient or family's opinion before they have had a chance to speak to an expert. However, it is also vital in the early stages of a complaint that you do not say anything negative about a medical colleague (even if you feel that they may have acted incorrectly). As a junior member of a team this would not be professional and should be dealt with by a senior doctor.

Question

How would you deal with a colleague who was not working as part of the team? (*250 words*)

This situation is one that is encountered in clinical practice and one that should be dealt with by the team leader. However, in many cases a junior member of the team who is not working well may cover their problems or mistakes and it may not get to the attention of a senior doctor. The panel want to know that you can find out what is going wrong and be professional about trying to remedy the situation.

Answer

The first thing that I would do would be to speak to my colleague in private. I would discuss any recent issues of clinical competency and ask if he or she had noticed any problems. I would also try and find out if there was any particular reason for a recent fall in productivity. There may be a personal problem that they need help with and I would try my best to help or otherwise direct them to people who I knew could help them. I would encourage them to review all problems in a positive light and see our conversation as a chance to improve the welfare of their patients.

If they were amenable, I would involve other junior members of the team to see if we could help them. It may be the case that after my interventions there were still difficulties. I would then approach another junior member of the team and explain the situation. If I felt that patient care was being compromised even after I had tried to help, I would have no hesitation in speaking to a senior member of the team. However, I would tell my colleague that I was going to do this and make sure that they understood that I was doing so only because patient care was paramount.

Question

What are your biggest weaknesses and how have you tried to change them in clinical practice? (200 words)

All doctors have areas of practice where they are less competent than they feel they should be. The panel want an honest answer to this question but also want you to show real evidence that you have tried to work on these weaknesses to better your clinical practice.

I think that my biggest weakness is that I take on too many responsibilities at once and this can sometimes lead to problems. For example, during my busy ST2 job in general surgery I decided to apply to sit on the hospital board of surgical consultants as the junior doctor representative for the year. This involved monthly meetings that I had to prepare for in terms of supervising audits, speaking to my colleagues about problems in the system and trying to improve patient care. In addition to these responsibilities I was also studying for my surgical MRCS exams and found that my performance in clinical teaching sessions was beginning to suffer.

I had to make the decision to drop my membership of the hospital board so that I could concentrate my free time on revising for my exams as I felt that this would be the best use of my time. I have learnt that rather than take on too may responsibilities at once it is far better to be absolutely sure that you can deal with current issues to the best of your ability. This is a skill that I am starting to learn and will try to improve as I continue my surgical training.

Question

What would you do if your consultant was being unfairly harsh to one of your colleagues on a ward round? (*200 words*)

Again, this question is one that is more often encountered in an interview but it has also been asked on application forms. Consultants can sometimes be demanding of their team and this expectation can in some cases cross the line to bullying. The panel want to know that you would try and identify a situation where this was occurring and help the junior member of staff. They need to see that you would respect the actions of your consultant on many cases but that if you really felt that bullying was occurring you would be able to deal with it appropriately.

Answer

The first thing I would do would be to speak to my colleague. I would make sure that he or she was well and not upset by the incident or incidents. I would do this in a quiet place away from other members of staff and I would tell them that any conversation between us would stay between the two of us unless they wanted me to speak to someone else. If my colleague had been performing less well than expected I would want to make sure there was no reason for this. They may have a professional or personal difficulty that I could help with.

If they felt that the consultant had acted harshly I would encourage them to speak to that consultant and explain that they had been upset by any comments directed at them. This should also take place in private away from other members of the team. If the consultant refused to discuss issues with my colleague or continued to act towards them in a difficult manner I would speak to another senior member of the team such as the SpR. I would have no hesitation in speaking to another consultant about the situation if I felt that there was a serious problem.

Feedback to the shortlisting process

If you are unsuccessful at any stage in the recruitment process, you have the right to request feedback from the deanery. Information about where to send your request will be available on the deanery's website. Your written request should state your full name, GMC number, specialty and level applied for. If you feel that your application process has been conducted unfairly, there is a complaints procedure in place within each deanery.

Applicants who write or phone for more specific feedback on their application form will be asked to meet with either their educational supervisor in the first instance or, if not readily available, someone who has previously and recently been involved in recruitment and selection for their specialty, who will be able to go through their form with them.

Any requests for further details other than those outlined earlier will be dealt with by deaneries under the Data Protection Act. Applicants who contact deaneries for their shortlisting scores should receive a copy of the following information:

- Rank and/or score
- Total number of applicants
- Rank and/or score required to gain an interview.

Example of a scoring system as used for specialty training

Table 5.1 is a real-life example of a scoring system as used by the London Deanery for specialty training shortlisting. This example is for academic

Table 5.1: Feedback to shortlisting process

	Essential	When evaluated	Desirable	When evaluated
Qualifications	Eligible for registration with the GMC	Application form	Intercalated BSc, BA, MSc	Application form
	MB BS (or equivalent)	Application form	Other degrees/ qualifications	Application form
	MRCS	Application form		
Clinical experience	3 years higher specialist training (or equivalent) by time of taking up post	Application form	ATLS/APLS/ ALS within 2 years	Application form
	Demonstrates competence in all core skills	Interview		
	Demonstrates educational progression supported by a satisfactory RITA Cs (attach to application form)	Interview		
Clinical skills	Competent to work without direct supervision where appropriate	Interview, reference		
	Clear, logical thinking showing an analytical/ scientific approach	Application form, interview		
	Good manual dexterity and hand/eye co-ordination	Reference		
Knowledge	Appropriate level of clinical knowledge	Reference	Demonstrates breadth of experience and awareness in and outside specialty/ medicine	Application form, interview

	Essential	When evaluated	Desirable	When evaluated
	Shows knowledge of evidence-informed practice	Interview	Demonstrates use of evidence-informed practice	Interview
	Shows awareness of own limitations	Interview, reference		
	Understanding of clinical risk management	Interview		
Organisation and planning	Ability to prioritise clinical need	Interview, reference	Understanding of NHS, clinical governance & resource constraints; management/ financial awareness; experience of committee work	Application form, interview
	Ability to organise oneself & work on own	Interview, reference		
	Evidence of participation and active involvement in an audit project	Application form, interview		
	Experience and ability to work in multi-professional teams	Application form, interview,	Information technology skills	Application form
Teaching skills	Evidence of teaching experience; involvement in organised teaching	Application form, interview	Enthusiasm for teaching; exposure to different groups/ teaching methods	Application form, interview
			Teaching the teachers course and certificate	Application form, interview

posts for applications for clinical lectureship positions but can be adapted to all specialty training posts. The essential criteria reflect objectives that all candidates must meet in full if they are to be considered for shortlisting. These include procedural objectives such as GMC registration and postgraduate exams in the specialty as well as specialty-specific criteria such as appropriate operating skills.

The desirable criteria are used to decide which candidates are to be called for interview and include extra-clinical qualifications such as ATLS exams and management skills such as the understanding of NHS Governance and formal teaching qualifications.

Sources of further information

NHS Foundation Programme: http://www.foundationprogramme.nhs.uk/

Modernising Medical Careers: http://www.mmc.nhs.uk/

Postgraduate Medical Education and Training Board (PMETB): http://www.pmetb.org.uk/

National recruitment office for GP training: http://www.gprecruitment.org.uk/

6

Specialty training interviews

Key aims of this chapter

- Give an idea of what to expect at interview
- Advise on how to prepare for the interview
- Discuss the different types of interview and detail commonly asked questions.

Introduction

Well done, you've made it as far the interview but it's not over quite yet. The interview requires an immense amount of preparation and should be treated as you would any other viva. It's not uncommon to see people come unstuck on the day, and this is purely due to a lack of preparation.

Most interviews are organised at deanery level, with a smaller variable number run by NHS Trusts, and typically more people are invited to interview than there are posts to ensure that all the jobs are filled. Once shortlisted, you should be notified of the date, time and location of the interview and this is usually done by e-mail (so keep an eye on your spam e-mail folder where deanery e-mails can sometimes go missing) but may also be by post. Details of the interviewing process and scoring scheme should be available to you at your request and you should aim to get an idea of the format well ahead of the interview day. This will guide your preparation.

You are typically given 5 days notice of the interview, however, it can be less, so if you are relatively confident that you will be shortlisted following the application, it is worthwhile noting the dates of the interviews for that specialty (found on the deanery website) and gently start to prepare.

You should also inform your current employer or colleagues of your potential interview dates, so they aren't left short on the day. Importantly, you will have a limited timeframe in which to confirm your intention to attend the interview and if you don't get an email back acknowledging your response, you should contact the deanery by telephone to confirm.

If you are lucky to be in the position where you have been interviewed and have accepted a job in a different post, you should out of courtesy let the deanery know and you will be withdrawn from the interview process; this will give someone else the opportunity to be interviewed. You should also inform the deanery if there is a clash of interview dates, for example, if you are invited to interview in two different specialties; where this occurs it may be possible to move interview times and dates but you need to give the deanery plenty of notice.

If you don't hear anything after your application has been sent in, this suggests that you have not been shortlisted for interview, as only successful candidates are contacted. However, it is worth contacting your centre of application (lead deanery or Royal College) if you think that perhaps the invitation for interview may have been 'lost'. If you think you have unfairly not been shortlisted, a complaints and appeals procedure is in place to deal with this type of query.

Pre-interview

A number of deaneries, e.g. Yorkshire Deanery, will offer mock interviews and it is worth contacting the deanery you have been shortlisted for to see if they offer such as service. Mock interviews are usually held either at the deanery or within education centres affiliated to the deanery. The earlier you ask about these opportunities the better, as places often fill up rapidly.

The interview is about demonstrating to the panel that not only do you meet the person specifications for the post, but that you are also the best person for the job. Your responses to questions should be structured and this means that potential questions should be thought through before the interview. You should ask colleagues, your educational supervisor and your consultant trainer for interview advice and more importantly, interview practice. Moreover, it is essential you ask for feedback as this will be the ideal opportunity for you to correct any annoying mannerisms or poor technique before the important day.

Interview day – what to take

You should receive information from your deanery as to what you should take to interview. The deanery is required to verify your identity, registration, qualifications and status with respect to working, and the following are usually required to do this. It is worth packing these well in advance of the day, along with any other documents requested:

- Proof of identity, e.g. passport or official photo ID (original plus two photocopies)
- Two recent, passport-type photographs with your name written clearly on the back of each
- Your original GMC certificate for the current year and two photocopies
- Your original degree certificate and relevant postgraduate qualifications including evidence of all qualifications listed on your application form, and including official translations if the original is not in English (original plus two photocopies)
- Evidence of educationally approved posts held as stated in your application form
- Verified evidence of competencies cited on your application form – i.e. your portfolio
- Evidence of eligibility to take up employment in the UK, including evidence of immigration status if a non-UK/EEA applicant, or an appropriate passport, birth certificate or naturalisation papers for UK/EEA applicants (plus two photocopies).

If for any reason you cannot provide the required documents you should provide a certified copy and contact the deanery prior to your interview, as failure to produce any of the requested documents may result in you not being interviewed.

It should be possible to claim travelling expenses for attending the interview. Expense forms should be available at interview and some deaneries ask for confirmation that you will be claiming for travel expenses in advance of the interview or require a request in writing, especially if overnight accommodation is required. Costs are paid in accordance with the Whitley Council Terms and Conditions, and receipts for costs incurred will need to be produced.

Box 6.1 Claiming travel expenses

Interview day – tips

First impressions in any interview count. Below is some general advice to help steer you away from trouble:

- Dress code for interviews is smart and conservative. Men should wear suits with ties and women similarly, should wear suits/jackets.
- Arrive early for the interview
  - If you are running late you should telephone through as it may be possible to reorganise the timings of the interview. If you just turn up late, then you may end up not being interviewed
  - If you are driving, make sure beforehand there are parking facilities available, and that you have enough change with you for the parking meter
  - If taking public transport, leave plenty of time for unexpected cancellations/delays
- Try not to make plans for after the interview. Interview schedules often run behind time, so if you need to be somewhere shortly after the interview, you are likely to be late.

Interview structure

The structure of interviews will vary across deaneries, specialties and your level of entry. Most postgraduate medical interviews are structured or semi-structured, which means that all candidates will be asked the same questions or questions with a similar theme, so it really is in your best interest not to divulge questions to candidates awaiting interview on the same day.

The number of stations can vary from anywhere between two to six, and within each station there will be usually be either two or three panel members. Generally, at ST/CT entry interviews will last for a minimum of 30 minutes, and each station will last a minimum of 10 minutes. You should expect to cover between three and four questions within each station.

Guidelines recommend that the interview panel should include the following members:

- A lay chair or lay representation, which can be a non-executive director, senior nurse, patient advocate, medical personnel representative or anyone not directly involved in training junior doctors or dentists.
- The regional college adviser or nominated deputy
- A university representative

- The programme director
- A consultant representative from the training programme(s)
- A senior management/human resources representative.

Before the interview, all members of the panel will have had access to your application form, excluding any equal opportunities or personal data. The interview panel members will have met with the lay chairman 30–45 minutes before the start of the interview. At this point interviewers will be allocated to their station, and will be in discussion with their panel co-members to determine what questions they are each going to ask.

The interview itself

- At the beginning of the interview the panel members will introduce themselves to you and will often offer you a handshake.
- Be positive and confident (not overconfident) – you have been invited to interview so you have a clear chance of securing the job.
- Listen carefully to the question asked and ensure that you understand the question.
  - If you don't understand the question, ask the interviewer to repeat the question – this should be done only once or twice during the interview as it can annoy some interviewers.
- Don't rush into answering a question. When you hear a question and if it is something that you can answer easily and you are prepared for, take a second or two before you start. It is often the first sentence that leads the discussion relating to that part of the interview and it is surprising how many people, even though they know that subject matter very well, start so badly that they are never able to recover.
- Answer the question! Don't go off on a tangent or answer the question that you would have liked them to ask you.
- Be honest in your response to questions. The panel are looking to employ a future colleague and enthusiasm, commitment and honesty are essential.
- Direct your response to the person asking the question, but make sure you don't ignore the other panel members.
- Avoid sounding as though you have rote-learnt answers to questions and even if you have a well-rehearsed response to a question, pause and deliver your reply as naturally as possible.
- In general:
  - If you are asked to give an opinion, it is useful to initially give both sides of the argument. However, don't sit on the fence. You will

undoubtedly be challenged and you should be able to defend your stance whilst demonstrating an ability to listen to other perspectives.

○ Where possible or appropriate you should try to demonstrate reflective practise, e.g. when asked to describe a situation, structure your response by giving some information regarding the setting, describe your involvement and the skills you called upon, and reflect on the outcome in terms of what you have learnt from the experience and how you may tackle the same or similar situation in the future.

○ Throughout the interview maintain good eye contact with all members of the panel.

○ Avoid fidgeting – place your hands firmly on your knees throughout the interview if this helps.

○ During the interview you may hear bells or knocks on the door indicating the times. Do not be put off by these. Keep talking until someone tells you that the interview has finished. If a question/station does go badly, try and put it behind you and importantly remain calm. The odds are you haven't done as badly as you feel you have.

● At the end of the interview, you may be asked whether you have any questions. You will not be penalised for not having any questions, so your options are:

○ Politely say no (the safest option)

○ Ask a question. Beware however that the question has not been answered elsewhere, e.g. in the person specification.

● At the termination of a station you will be asked by the coordinator to wait and then will be directed to the next station.

● At the end of the interview, remember to thank the interviewer(s) and don't leave anything behind.

● Once you have finished all of the stations you will be allowed to leave the interview room.

Marking the candidate

In each station each panel member will mark the sections discussed in that station separate to co-panel members according to the person specification for the post, and have the opportunity to add comments to justify the score given. There will therefore be two sets of marks at least for each station.

After the interviews have been completed, all the marks for each of the candidates are collated and added up and, as a result of this, the candidates are ranked. It is not possible for the marks to be changed as they are collected from the panel members by the administrative coordinator at regular intervals during the interviews and are collated into the accumulated scores. In the briefing discussion before the interviews begin, the panel members may decide that certain questions are so important that should the candidate not answer them correctly they will be 'red carded'. This often relates to clinical scenarios where the panel may feel that the candidate's clinical experience, if they could not answer the question appropriately, would deem them unsuitable for the post for which they were being interviewed.

The panel members and the lay chairman before the interview discuss the issue of 'red carding' and establish clear guidelines as to the grounds on which a red card can be issued. After the interview, when the marks are looked at, although a candidate may have been ranked high enough to be offered a job, if they have been 'red carded' in any section of the interview, they will be automatically eliminated from the selection.

Role of references at interview

References can be unstructured (free-text) or be structured. In the latter your referee may be asked a number of questions including those regarding your clinical ability, future potential, team-working skills and interaction with patients and colleagues – those attributes as outlined by the GMC's document *Good Medical Practice*. The references are not seen by the panel members but are viewed only by the lay chairman. A key role of the lay chairman is to review the written references, to ensure that there is nothing in the reference that would deem the person unappointable. References will also be reviewed by the employer if you are successful at interview.

Types of question at interview

The interview panel will essentially be looking for specific qualities as stated in the person specification for the post, and this will be achieved through assessment over a number of stations, and each station which look at a different skill sets. As part of your interview preparation you should consider questions that are commonly asked and prepare answers to each according to your own personal experiences. Below are the key areas likely to be assessed:

Clinical knowledge and expertise

- Appropriate knowledge base
- Capacity to apply sound clinical judgement to problems
- Ability to prioritise clinical need
- Aware of the basics of managing acutely ill patients.

Vigilance and situational awareness

- Capacity to be alert to dangers or problems
- Capacity to monitor developing situations and anticipate issues.

Coping with pressure

- Capacity to operate under pressure
- Initiative and resilience to cope with setbacks and adapt to rapidly changing circumstances
- Awareness of own limitations and when to ask for help.

Managing others and team involvement

- Capacity to work cooperatively with others
- Ability to work effectively in multiprofessional teams
- Leadership skills.

Problem solving and decision making

- Capacity to solve problems
- Ability to make decisions.

Empathy and sensitivity

- Capacity to take in others' perspectives and treat others with understanding
- Sees patients as people.

Communication skills

- Demonstrates clarity in written/spoken communication
- Adapts language as appropriate to the situation
- Able to build rapport, listen, persuade and negotiate.

Organisation and planning

- Capacity to organise oneself, prioritise own work and organise ward rounds

- Demonstrates punctuality, preparation and self-discipline
- Possesses basic IT skills.

Professional integrity and respect for others

- Capacity to take responsibility for own actions
- Demonstrates a non-judgemental approach towards others
- Displays honesty, integrity, awareness of confidentiality and ethical issues
- Possesses delegation skills.

Learning and personal development

- Demonstrates interest and realistic insight specialty
- Demonstrates self-awareness
- Ability to accept feedback
- Extracurricular activities/achievements relevant to acute medicine.

There can be a great variation in the type of stations encountered at interview but they will usually include two or more of the following:

1. Portfolio-based interviews
2. Research, teaching and publications
3. Clinical governance, audit and management
4. Clinical experience
5. Behavioural/situational questions – these are aimed at addressing aspects of the person specification such as team working, ethics etc.
6. Communications station
7. Presentations
8. Assessment of practical or examination skills.

1. Portfolio-based interviews

At ST1/CT1 portfolio-based stations are commonplace and can be used to assess a number of aspects of your person specification including your career progression and learning and development. Within these stations you may simply be asked to hand over your portfolio for review by the examiner or you may be asked questions centred on your portfolio. The aim of questioning in this context is to substantiate the evidence contained within your portfolio and to assess your motivation to the specialty you are applying to. This is your to opportunity to shine. You should know your portfolio inside out.

- A list of competencies required to successfully complete the foundation programme
- Records of meetings with your educational supervisor
- A PDP including career planning
- Presented evidence
  - Exam certificates
  - Certificates of course/lecture/tutorial attendance
  - Posters presented at learned meetings
  - Presentations including at journal clubs
  - Abstracts and papers (full texts)
  - Audit projects (full texts)
  - A reflective log of activities and experience
  - A logbook of clinical activity or record of achieved competencies signed by your trainer, e.g. procedures or operations
- WBAs
  - 360-degree assessments or mini-PATS
  - DOPs
  - Mini-CEX
  - CBDs
  - PBAs

Box 6.2 Inclusions for your logically presented portfolio for the interview

A common opening question is, 'Talk me through your portfolio.' Although this should be straightforward, it is also a very easy question to answer badly. Remember that you only have a limited amount of time, so try and structure your answer, demonstrating focus in your career pathway to date, commitment to your specialty and drive. You should summarise your clinical experience and highlight your strengths and achievements; you should also outline where you see yourself in the near future.

Other frequently asked questions include: (1) 'What have you learnt whilst putting together your portfolio?', (2) 'Why do you think it is important to maintain a portfolio?' and (3) 'What are your strengths and weaknesses as evidenced by your portfolio?'

Other questions may be aimed at establishing your commitment to the specialty or deanery you have applied to, for example: (1) 'Why have you applied to this deanery?', (2) 'How have you demonstrated your commitment and aptitude for this specialty?', (3) 'What have you done outside of your

regular schedule that demonstrates your interest in this specialty?',
(4) 'What qualities are needed for a career in this particular specialty?' and
(5) 'Why this specialty?' The former may be evidenced by previous posts
held, 'tasters', membership of the relevant learned societies, attendance
of courses or meetings relevant to your specialty and specialty-specific
research/audit and these should be brought out in the interview.

2. Research, teaching and publications

At CT/ST entry level it is unlikely you will encounter an individual Research,
Teaching and Publications station, since your experience in this area at
this point is likely to be limited. Questions on teaching, research and
publications may however be covered elsewhere in the interview, such as
your portfolio station. The obvious exception to this is application for posts
in academic medicine.

Research

Discussion in this part of the interview will centre on any academic research
that you have previously conducted or are currently performing. You may
have completed an intercalated BSc or a BSc before entering medical school.
Others may have done an MSc, performed research as part of their elective
or even completed an MBPhD.

A common opening question is: 'Tell us about your research experience
or any research you have conducted.' With any question at interview, you
should pause and give a structured response to the question, instead of
rushing into an answer. Here, a chronological and clear description of your
experience to date is expected and you should be prepared to answer
questions on your research. For example, if you mention laboratory-based
research you may be asked about laboratory methods and statistics used.
In addition, you should be prepared to answer research-related questions,
such as: (1) 'How has this research impacted on clinical practice?' or (2)
'What have you gained from your research?'

Publications

Presentations and publications will, in the main, be derived from research
or audit you have conducted, individual case reports or clinical reviews.
When completing the application form you should read the section on
publications very carefully. Although it may fill the space on the form, to

list publications including abstracts and letters or papers that are either in progress or submitted, can irritate some interviewers. At interview, interviewers will want to know about the publications that have actually been accepted or published.

Common questions in this area are: (1) 'Out of all of your publications, which one is the most important?' or (2) 'Which one have you made the greatest contribution to?' When answering this question, you should acknowledge to the panel the level of your contribution, and even if you have not performed all of the work yourself, you should have a clear understanding of all parts of paper, e.g. methods of cell culture, RNA extraction etc. Other associated questions that may arise include those on evidenced-based medicine, such as: (1) 'What is evidence-based medicine?' or (2) 'Do you practice evidence-based medicine?' and those on research methodology, for example, (1) 'What do you understand by levels of evidence?', (2) 'What do you understand by the term "randomised control trial" (RCT)?', (3) 'How do you set up a research project and a clinical trial?' etc. Questions regarding basic statistics are also not uncommon, e.g. (1) 'What is sensitivity and specificity?' or (2) 'What is statistical power?' etc.

Teaching

By this point in your career, you are unlikely to have formal teaching experience. At interview a common opening question is: 'Tell us what experience you have of teaching.'

Most people will have had experience of teaching undergraduates, and this may be lecturing on revision courses and preparing medical students for their exams or teaching during their attachment on your firm. A few interviewees may also have experience of teaching postgraduates, e.g. colleagues, and other healthcare professionals. For instance, nurses, physiotherapists, ambulance crews etc. Your teaching experience may also extend to developing or organising postgraduate and undergraduate courses, and it is essential that you make sure you discuss these in detail during the interview. It is also useful when answering this question to give some idea of your time commitment to teaching, for example, you may teach medical students for 2 hours each week.

Questions following from this may require discussion of your own teaching strengths or weaknesses, your preferred teaching methods and the attributes of a good teacher. Importantly, teaching experience is not just about delivering teaching but it is also about developing teaching skills.

You may have attended a course, such as Teaching the Teachers, or have undertaken an intercalated medical education degree, which you should bring into the discussion.

3. Clinical governance, audit and management

Clinical governance

In this station, clinical governance will often be dealt with using clinical case scenarios, and the example used will be different for different specialties. An example in surgery may be: 'What do you do if a swab has been left in the wound and the swab count is incorrect at the end of the procedure?' In general medicine, similar scenarios may relate to your management of patients who have been given the wrong medication; either the wrong drug or the wrong dose, or a drug interaction. For example: 'A patient who has a penicillin allergy is accidentally administered penicillin. How would tackle this?', or 'How do you explain to a patient that a postoperative complication has arisen?'

The GMC gives clear guidance within *Good Medical Practice* regarding the management of adverse events at work:

"If a patient under your care has suffered harm or distress, you must act immediately to put matters right, if that is possible. You should offer an apology and explain fully and promptly to the patient what has happened, and the likely short-term and long-term effects... Patients who complain about the care or treatment they have received have a right to expect a prompt, open, constructive and honest response including an explanation and, if appropriate, an apology. You must not allow a patient's complaint to affect adversely the care or treatment you provide or arrange."

Box 6.3 *Good Medical Practice* advice on handling adverse events

All of these types of clinical scenarios also require you to mention critical incident reporting and you should be prepared to answer related questions, such as: (1) 'What happens to the clinical incident form after you have completed it?', (2) 'What feedback is given as a result of a clinical incident?' and (3) 'Give an example where the outcome of action you took in response to a clinical mistake/error made you reassess how you would deal with similar events in the future.' In this station you should also be prepared to give a definition of clinical governance and an example of where it has proved important to you and changed your practice.

Audit

You should have either initiated or been involved in an audit by this stage in your career. Audit questions will usually start along the line of: (1) 'What is audit?,' (2) 'Discuss one of the audits that you have done,' (3) 'Tell me about your most interesting audit,' or (4) 'Tell me about the audit that you think is most valuable.'

You will be expected to discuss an audit or audits that you have undertaken, why you undertook them, what results you obtained and, of course, what has been done to close the loop and the impact of the audit on your clinical practice. Further questions may include: (1) 'What is clinical audit?,' (2) 'What are the benefits of audit?' and (3) 'How does audit differ from research?'

Management

Management for junior trainees is a difficult topic to discuss at interview since most foundation trainees will have had little experience of management at this stage. In this part of the interview, discussions on management are far more likely to focus on specific areas such as NICE, European Working Time Directive (EWTD), MMC etc. For example: (1) 'What is NICE?,' (2) 'Describe one NICE guideline in relation to your specialty?,' (3) 'Is it possible to train in a 48-hour week?,' (4) 'What do you understand by the Hospital at Night (H@N) scheme?' and (5) 'What is the World Health Organisation (WHO) checklist in surgery and what are its components?'

4. Clinical knowledge and expertise

The aim of this part of the interview is to determine your suitability for entry at CT1/ST1. The interviewers will have a copy of your application form, and as an opening question you may be asked to discuss your clinical experience to date. In these types of questions, the interviewer does not want to hear a list of hospitals and dates of when you worked there. Instead, you need to take them through your personal story, and you may be asked to discuss one or two jobs in more critical detail.

One approach would be to discuss all the positive things that you have gained from each of your posts and if a particular post was weak in one area you should acknowledge this, but also draw on how you addressed this.

For example: 'My exposure to x was poor in this post, however in my next job there was more than ample opportunity to remedy this deficiency in my training.' This makes it appear that you are planning your career sensibly.

Other questions in this section will often be related to clinical scenarios. There are a huge number of clinical scenarios that can arise and they will depend upon the specialty to which you are applying. Most scenarios are based upon real incidents and during this station the interviewers are looking to see if you are safe and whether you have had hands-on experience or the skills necessary to cope with your level of entry into specialist training. Moreover, they want to determine whether you are going to be a coherent, sensible voice at the end of the phone at 2am.

Often the scenarios will relate to the management of a medical or surgical emergency, such as managing an acute exacerbation of asthma, massive gastrointestinal (GI) bleed, an acutely ischaemic limb, torsion of the testis, postoperative bleeding or a trauma patient brought into 'resus'. Alternatively, scenarios may be based around cases commonly encountered in either an Accident and Emergency (A & E department), ward or outpatient setting, for example, management of an elderly patient with iron-deficiency anaemia, management of a postoperative patient with pyrexia or sudden-onset shortness of breath or management of an 85-year-old diabetic with a 5-day history of vomiting and abdominal pain.

Other scenarios may relate to practical procedures, such as insertion of a central venous pressure catheter, or even male catheterisation. You may also be asked to describe basic operations, such as excision of a sebaceous cyst or inguinal hernia repair; this is especially true if this has been listed in your logbook. In the weeks before interview you should prepare by going through clinical cases that you have seen or ones that you believe may be important to the specialty you are applying to.

At interview, you need to listen carefully to the clinical scenario, as the wording will often give you clues as to what the interviewer is trying to probe from you. Remember with clinical scenarios that although there is often more than one way to deal with the case, the fundamentals will remain the same. Management means resuscitating the patient, taking a history, examining the patient, formulating a differential diagnosis, investigating the patient, establishing a definitive diagnosis and treating the patient. Importantly, you should also demonstrate a multidisciplinary approach to the patient's care involving other specialists (e.g. radiologists, neurosurgeons, anaesthetists) and your seniors/consultant as appropriate. You should not be afraid to ask for help.

Throughout this station, you should demonstrate a logical approach and demonstrate a clear understanding of the management of the condition in your answer. If you really don't know, rather than make things up, you should say you don't know, but would seek advice from senior colleagues. Additionally, if you forget something important in a patient's management, you should acknowledge this. Furthermore, do not allow long silences while you try and think of your next step. It is much better to say that you have forgotten or that you do not know and to move onto the next topic rather than to just sit there in silence. It will usually be quite apparent to the panel members that this is just a short memory lapse.

Other questions in this station may be designed to test a combination of qualities as defined in the person specification. For example: 'You have two patients in A & E admitted at the same time. One with a suspected ruptured abdominal aortic aneurysm, a second with a gastric perforation and your FY1 is concerned about a patient on the ward who is unwell. How would you tackle the situation?' This scenario requires you to demonstrate good communication skills, team working and leadership, as well as the ability to keep calm under pressure, and rapidly assess, prioritise and recognise sick patients. Importantly, in these scenarios, you are not expected to be in more than one place at the same time. However, by using effective communication and calling for help early as well as delegating tasks this scenario may be managed successfully with no detrimental effect on patient care.

Further questions in this section may be geared towards gauging your understanding of clinical processes. For example, a trainee surgeon could be asked about the personnel in theatre or about the WHO checklist in surgery.

5. Behavioural questions

Other qualities in the person specification may be assessed using situational or behavioural questions, in addition to, or as part of more generic questions.

Work-related behavioural or situational questions are becoming increasingly more popular in medicine and are used to assess your performance in the past, the theory being that past performance is often the best predictor of future performance in a similar situation. Situational questions are thought to be more objective than traditional questions and following an often very open-ended starting question, the interviewer can then probe deeper with further questions, e.g. 'How did you feel at the time?'

Although the number of potential situational questions that could arise is exhaustive, it is useful to think of a handful of scenarios beforehand that can be adapted to cover the most common questions or that demonstrate the necessary key person-specific qualities. Each answer should be specific and incorporate some background/scene-setting information (this should be brief), the specific action you took (which demonstrates a specific quality within the person specification) and the positive outcome. An example of a situational question would be: 'Describe a time when you have had to co-ordinate the activities of a team in a critical situation and how you dealt with the stress?' This question assesses both your ability to cope with stress as well as manage others within a team and problem solve. You should use 'real' examples in your response, and avoid embellishing the truth.

Other so-called generic questions may more specifically target one aspect of the person specification. For example, to assess your 'vigilance and situational awareness', you may be asked to: 'Describe an example from your experience in this specialty when applying your clinical judgment had a defining impact on patient management. What did you do and how do you think the outcome was affected by your judgement?' To assess your ability to team-work, you may be asked: (1) 'How do you ensure good teamwork?,' (2) 'What is a team and why is teamwork important?' or (3) 'Give an example where you showed leadership.' Although, as a junior doctor, you are not expected to have developed the same level of leadership skills as your more senior colleagues, applicants should be able to demonstrate a clear understanding of the attributes that make a good leader and be seen to be starting to develop these skills.

In relation to other components of the person specification, to assess your 'problem solving and decision making' you may be asked: (1) 'How do you deal with a patient who presents with a condition that you are unfamiliar with?' or (2) 'What do you do if the night F2 does not turn up for his shift?'. To assess your 'organisation and planning' skills, you may be asked: 'How do you effectively organise your day?' and so forth.

Difficult interview questions

Difficult interview questions often draw on multiple aspects of the person specification. A good example is those relating to conflict at work; this may be a conflict with a colleague, e.g. a senior doctor who refuses to review a sick patient, other healthcare professionals, e.g. a nurse who disagrees with your management plan, or a relative who is unhappy with a family member's care and is quite aggressive. Conflict-type questions are common and need careful preparation but the answer will inevitably involve communication skills, negotiation and initiative, empathy, teamworking and possibly also clinical incidence reporting. You must emphasise that you will listen to the views of all of those involved in the altercation, and then negotiate some form of mutually acceptable resolution to the conflict.

Other difficult questions may centre on colleagues in difficulty. For example: 'How do you manage a colleague who is working under the influence of alcohol or drugs?'

Importantly, you should remember that you have a duty of care to you patient. *Good Medical Practice* clearly states, "You must protect patients from risk of harm posed by another colleague's conduct, performance or health. The safety of patients must come first at all times. If you have concerns that a colleague may not be fit to practise, you must take appropriate steps without delay so that the concerns are investigated and patients protected where necessary."

Box 6.4 Duty of care

It is important to appreciate here that 'difficult' doctors, may themselves be in difficulty, i.e. they may be under work (conflict with colleagues/managers) or personal pressure (domestic, financial, bereavement), ill, not coping (physically or mentally), insecure, inadequately trained, lacking in motivation etc. There are a number of avenues available to you to resolve this matter. Local systems should be in place, and you should initially attempt to seek local resolution.

If you feel you can, it may be appropriate to talk directly to the doctor involved. If not, you should contact an appropriate lead within your Trust, e.g. clinical director, educational supervisor, senior clinician or deanery. Where local mechanisms fail, you should consider contacting the GMC.

6. Assessment of communication skills at interview

Your communication skills will be continuously assessed throughout the course of the interview and you should be aware of your body language, and language throughout the day.

Communication skills can also be more formally assessed within a communications station. This may involve role-playing with the use of actors/patients or the interviewer. Common scenarios encountered include:

● Consent for a procedure such as colonoscopy
● Breaking bad news, e.g. to a patient with cancer

- Dealing with difficult patients, e.g. a patient who refuses treatment and wishes to self-discharge
- Dealing with difficult colleagues
- A telephone call to your consultant, e.g. to discuss patients admitted on-call
- An outpatient consultation.

Good communication (i.e. listening, negotiation and compromise to reach resolution) is usually the mainstay for management of these scenarios.

The GMC's document, *Good Medical Practice* (2006) gives guidelines regarding effectively communicating with patients, stating you should:

- "Listen to patients,
- Ask for and respect their views
- Respond to their concerns and preferences
- Share with patients, in a way they can understand, the information they want or need to know about their condition, it's likely progression, and the treatment options available to them, including associated risks and uncertainties
- Respond to patients' questions and keep them informed about the progress of their care
- Make sure that patients are informed about how information is shared within teams and among those who will be providing their care
- You must make sure, wherever practical, that arrangements are made to meet patients' language and communication needs."

Box 6.5 Patient communication

7. Assessing presentation skills at interview

Communication may be assessed at interview by asking you to give a presentation (this may or may not be pre-planned). Some interviews will merely assess the overall style of presentation but others will mark the content as well.

If pre-planned, you will usually be advised of the topic of the presentation at the time of notification of the interview. Presentations will be expected in PowerPoint format, and topics are varied and can be medical/clinical (where the emphasis is often on audit, medical ethics or the multidisciplinary approach to patient care) or non-medical, where the emphasis is often on topics such as team building, management, problem solving and communication skills.

Alternatively, you may be asked just prior to going into the interview to make a two or three-minute presentation and you may or may not be allowed to use visual aids – this will usually be in the form of a single overhead transparency. The questions are likely to be generic here, e.g. (1) 'Why are you the best person for the job?,' (2) 'Why have you chosen this specialty?' or (3) 'Describe your strengths and weaknesses.' The purpose of this second type of presentation in addition to assessing your communication and presentation skills is to assess your ability to think on your feet and to be dynamic.

All shortlisted candidates will be given the same topic, so the panel may very well have heard the same or similar presentation several times over by the time yours is heard. Try and make your presentation different, but most of all keep to time, as you may be cut short if you don't.

General tips on preparing presentations

- Your presentation should be in Microsoft PowerPoint and in landscape mode
- Your first slide should contain the presentation title and your name only
- Do not overcrowd your slides; ideally there should be no more than 4–5 bullet points or 9–15 words per slide
- As a rule of thumb, you should expect to take 30–40 seconds per slide (may be up to 2 minutes for more complex slides) and you should adjust your total number of slides to your time limit
- Choose the size of your font carefully – ideally it should be 28 pt or greater
- Avoid using a busy or distracting background, i.e. stick to a plain or non-offensive slide background
- Choose your text and background colours carefully and try and avoid reds and greens as your interviewers may be colour blind
- Avoid excess animation and focus on the content of your presentation; now is not the time to work on getting laughs
- Don't simply read your slides – the bullets on the slides should merely be a prompt and summary of the salient points. Keep it simple
- Speak clearly and confidently and make eye-contact with the interviewers
- Pace the presentation – don't suddenly realise in the last 30 seconds that you still have a third of the presentation left to go through
- Practice your presentation and if possible do this in front of friends or colleagues and get them to ask questions and comment on ways that you could improve your presentation

- You must make sure that you keep to time
- When delivering your presentation, watch where you stand and ensure you don't obscure or detract attention from your slides
- If you are likely to need a laser-pointer you must take one along with you to the interview as one may not always be available
- Draw up a list of the possible questions that you may be asked in relation to the topic on which you are presenting and be prepared to answer these
- When answering questions, don't be defensive or argumentative
- Bring a back-up copy of your presentation, e.g. on an additional memory stick.

Where you are only given a short period of time to prepare a presentation, the same general principles as above can be applied. Importantly, the interviewers will expect you to be nervous, so don't worry if you stutter or the presentation doesn't quite go to plan.

8. Assessment of practical skills at interview

An additional station may be present in some interviews that is designed specifically to assess practical ability. This is more likely to be present in the craft specialties and will, generally speaking, involve quite simple tasks such as suturing and tying knots, and inserting a urinary catheter. Some skills may require familiarity with commonly used instruments in that specialty. For instance, in otolaryngology, familiarity with an otoscope would be an important practical skill.

Finally, be prepared to conduct a systems examination (e.g. abdominal, vascular, neck, hip/knee etc.) on a mock patient; further discussions may then ensue regarding your management of the patient.

After the interview

When you go to the interview, you should check that the recruiting office has your correct contact details should you be made an offer, and you should also advise them of any reason or period of time when you may not be contactable.

Offers of posts to training programmes will be offered to interviewees who are ranked the highest at interview, and once given this offer you will have a limited amount of time, a minimum of 48 hours to accept or decline the offer, after which the offer will be withdrawn. If this is the best offer on the table, you should accept it as soon as possible and it is often wise to telephone your deanery to ensure they have received your email of acceptance.

At the same time you should decline any other offers you may also have, as these can be offered to other applicants. If you have accepted a job offer previously, you cannot accept a second offer, and offers are made by deaneries on the condition that you have not previously accepted any other post. The exceptions to this rule are Academic Clinical Fellowships and FTSTA posts. If you don't have any other offers on the table, you need to think carefully before declining an offer.

Once you have accepted a training programme, the deanery will match you to a specific post/rotation within the programme, and should advise you of the following:

- The name of your employer
- The start date and length (or likely length) of the period of employment
- The name of the position needing to be filled and the work needing to be done
- The location of the work
- The hours needing to be worked
- Any potential health and safety risks
- The qualifications/experience required to do the job
- Any expenses payable (e.g. removal/relocation)
- The minimum rate of remuneration payable and any other benefits on offer
- The intervals at which you will be paid
- The notice period applicable.

Once employment checks are successfully completed, and these include verification of references, fitness to practice updates from the GMC, occupational health clearance, CRB disclosures and immigration status checks, as a minimum, your new employer will confirm the post. You should receive your contract within 2 months of starting in post, as per NHS Employers' guidance.

What if you don't get a post?

You will be contacted by email if you are unsuccessful at interview and you should contact (write or email) your recruiting office to request feedback regarding your performance at interview and to seek careers advice. You will be sent your rank and/or score, the rank/score required to receive an offer, and the total number of applicants interviewed by the deanery.

You can also request copies of your interview score sheets. This should help guide your preparation for future interviews. In addition, you also need to assess whether the specialty and deanery you have chosen is realistic.

Importantly, you may still have a shot of the post you want, as deaneries will continue to advertise training vacancies beyond the first and second rounds throughout the year as they arise.

Sources of further information

Postgraduate Medical Education and Training Board (PMETB): http://www.pmetb.org.uk
GP training: http://gprecruitment.oth.uk
Recruitment to medical specialty training in Scotland: http://www.mmc.scot.nhs.uk
Recruitment to medical specialty training in Wales: http://www.mmcwales.org
Recruitment to medical specialty training in Northern Ireland: http://www.nimdta.gov.uk
Academic posts: http://www.nihrtcc.nhs.uk

7

GP recruitment

Key aims of this chapter

- Outline the process of GP recruitment in the UK
- Suggest ways in which candidates may prepare for this process
- Provide links to resources for preparation, and where appropriate, examples of the assessment methods used.

Introduction

Since 2006, the recruitment to GP training has moved from a traditional interview format to two assessments. Candidates who perform well in the first assessment will then be invited to attend the second. The purpose of these assessments is to provide a fair and evidence-based assessment of candidates for GP training in the UK, and all candidates will be assessed against the National Person Specification for GP training.

Part 1: Multiple matching test

The first assessment is an invigilated multiple matching test. Performance in this test forms part of the short-listing process. This first assessment is conducted on 1 day in deaneries across the UK and you should be able to attend at your closest available centre. You will have opportunity to select these through a central booking system. The assessment itself consists of two papers, one on professional dilemmas and the second on clinical problem solving. These papers are designed to assess the essential competencies as outlined in the National Person Specification, which is available from the official GP recruitment website.

Professional dilemmas paper

The duration of examination for this paper is 2 hours and it presents scenarios you might find in clinical practice. Each scenario encapsulates a professional dilemma. The paper is designed to assess your understanding of appropriate behaviour for a doctor in difficult situations. It tests the application of competencies such as professional integrity, coping with pressure, and empathy and sensitivity. It does not require specific knowledge of general practice beyond a broad knowledge of UK medical practice. At the time of writing, the favoured answer format is that of multiple ranked answers. Your responses should be appropriate for an FY2 doctor, and your score is based on how close your responses are to the most appropriate response as determined by a panel of expert GPs.

Clinical problem-solving paper

The duration for this paper is 90 minutes and it presents clinical scenarios that require you to exercise problem-solving skills to determine the appropriate diagnosis and management. This is not so much a test of knowledge, but rather the ability to apply it. The topics will be taken from areas with which an FY2 doctor should be familiar, and there are no questions requiring a specific knowledge of general practice. Questions may be presented in a variety of multiple matching formats, such as extended matching questions (EMQs) and single best answers (SBAs).

Preparation for papers

These papers have been introduced relatively recently as part of the selection process into general practice, however there is already a small industry producing practice questions. A number of sample questions are also available on the official GP recruitment website with full explanations; practice question books are also available from a number of publishers.

If there are obvious gaps in your knowledge then you need to address this before the assessment. Practising 'data interpretation' and 'situational judgement'-type questions may help you to identify these gaps in knowledge and re-familiarise you with multiple matching formats; this will also allow you to perfect your MCQ/SBA/EMQ technique.

There is no formally endorsed preparation book or course, however reading books such as the Oxford Handbook of Clinical Specialties, The Oxford Handbook of the Foundation Years will not do any harm. It is also worth being familiar with the General Medical Council document *Good Medical Practice* (2006).

On the day – advice on performing well in the multiple matching test

- Papers are not negatively marked so you should answer all of the questions
- Read the instructions and questions carefully as your answer may be invalidated by responding inappropriately
- There may be times when you would like more information to answer questions but it is best to just give your best answer given the information provided as all candidates will be in the same situation
- Where questions use terms or abbreviations that are not in universal use or may be misunderstood by some candidates, a glossary is provided in the examination and you should ask the invigilator if a term or abbreviation fitting this description is included within the glossary.

Part 2: Selection assessment centre

If you achieve the standard required at the first assessment you will be invited to a selection assessment centre (SAC). This will usually be at your first-choice deanery, although this will depend on the availability of places. You will only be invited to attend at one deanery. Your application will be considered for a training programme at the deanery where you attend the selection centre.

At each UK SAC candidates will be required to complete three exercises, each of which will be observed and assessed by trained assessors. The exercises will consist of a patient simulation exercise, a group exercise and a written exercise. There are no interviews and assessors do not have access to your application form, or any other biographical information. Assessors will look for the demonstration of evidence in the competency areas as described in the person specification and each candidate has a number of opportunities to demonstrate these.

What to expect on the day

Once you have registered, you will have your photograph taken. This is to ensure that the assessors can identify you during the selection process. You will be asked to indicate your preferred geographical areas or programmes within the deanery from those available and this will be explained when you attend. There will be a briefing session at the start of your SAC session and an opportunity for questions at the end of it. Individual feedback on your performance will only be given after the offers have been made.

What must I bring?

- Deaneries will request that references for all applicants who are invited to attend are brought on the day
- You will also be asked to provide photographic proof of identity such as a passport or driving licence
- You will be asked to provide documentation relating to your right to work in the UK
- Your original GMC certificate (and a photocopy)
- Your original medical qualification certificate (and a photocopy)
- If you do not currently hold a driving licence, you will be asked to confirm that you have suitable arrangements for attending emergencies and providing domiciliary care
- Originals of the evidence you submitted to demonstrate achievement of foundation competency for verification.

Patient simulation exercise

This will involve a simulator and a situation that you should be able to deal with as a doctor with at least 18 months' postgraduate experience. It will not involve a physical examination and clinical expertise is not specifically assessed. The following information details the candidate and actor's briefing packs for a typical patient simulation scenario:

Example scenario

You are the FY2 doctor in general practice.

Recent medical history:

Mr Peter Pevensey came a week ago with vague abdominal discomfort. Blood taken at that time showed a mild anaemia, high MCV and a raised gamma-GT.

Reason for consultation today:

The patient is coming in to discuss the results of the blood tests, which you will tell him. Mr Pevensey is tired-looking, unkempt and smells of alcohol. Please discuss his lifestyle and agree the next steps.

Actor's briefing:

You are a businessman who is feeling tired and washed-out so you had a blood test. You have come for the results. Though initially you deny having a drinking excess alcohol problem you are prepared to continue a dialogue.

If asked:

● You have a drink with most meals
● If pushed to answer, a drink means a bottle of wine (even if alone)
● You have occasionally failed to get to work the next day due to a hangover
● You occasionally will 'take the hair of the dog' and have a morning drink
● You did consider cutting down a few months ago, but then it was the run up to Christmas
● You sometimes feel guilty, especially when relatives have a go
● You find it really irritating when people badger you about drinking too much
● You have occasionally found yourself in situations you would not have chosen (you refuse to elaborate) as a result of being drunk
● You consider Alcoholics Anonymous a 'bit of a joke' and have confidentiality concerns
● You have no idea about units of alcohol
● If they ask you if you would be interested in finding out more about units of alcohol, cutting down and perhaps having a repeat test, you are more amenable
● If asked any specific questions not addressed in the briefing, please answer 'No'.

Tasks to achieve in this scenario

Consider how you would use the above case to demonstrate the following checklist:

● **Clinical knowledge and expertise:** Capacity to apply sound clinical knowledge and awareness to full investigation of problems
● **Empathy and sensitivity:** Capacity and motivation to take in others' perspectives and to treat others with understanding
● **Communication skills:** Capacity to adjust behaviour and language as appropriate to the needs of differing situations
● **Conceptual thinking and problem solving:** Capacity to think beyond the obvious, with an analytical and flexible mind
● **Coping with pressure:** Capacity to recognise own limitations and develop appropriate coping mechanisms
● **Organisation and planning:** Capacity to organise information/time effectively in a planned manner

- **Managing others and team involvement:** Capacity to work effectively in partnership with others.

Written exercise

This an exercise in which there are no absolutely correct answers. The assessors expect you to demonstrate your abilities against the competency areas identified in the person specification. Be familiar with this.

Example scenario

Your task (30 minutes):

The various issues listed below are presented to you on arrival and need to be prioritised for action. This should involve three stages:

1. Ranking each issue in the order in which you intend to deal with it
2. Justifying your decisions
3. Commenting on interesting and/or difficult challenges posed by the exercise:

   - All rankings, justifications and comments should be entered and completed within the appropriate boxes (see answer sheet).
   - For the first 5 minutes you should not write, but should study the challenge posed. You will be advised when you may start writing.
   - For the next 20 minutes you should complete the first two stages of the task listed earlier (ranking the issues and justifying your decisions).
   - For the final 5 minutes you should complete the third stage of the task (reflecting on the exercise).

Note that you will not be reminded about the time you have left. Issues to be ranked:

- The GP receptionist reminds you that there is a wheezy and slightly breathless patient who has been sitting in the waiting room for 2 hours, and has not yet been assessed by a doctor.
- The practice manager tells you that your mother has just phoned sounding very upset, and asking that you contact her urgently.
- An angry local has just come into the surgery complaining that your car is blocking access to his driveway and must be moved immediately.
- An FY2 doctor telephones from the local hospital. He says that the patient you felt was not coping at home has had his urinary infection treated and will be discharged home in the late afternoon.
- The receptionist reminds you that you are due to present the audit figures at the practice meeting, which starts in 10 minutes' time.

Group exercise

You will be randomly allocated to a group to carry out an exercise that will involve a group discussion; this will obviously involve interaction with colleagues and candidates going through the same selection process for a GP specialty training programme. The group dynamics are not assessed. The person specification is again the reference for assessors.

Preparation
- Visit the official GP recruitment website and read ALL the information. Of particular importance is the National Person Specification, which should be discussed with colleagues.
- Practice the example scenarios with your colleagues.
- Read *Good Medical Practice* (GMC 2006) and consider discussing how the duties of a doctor may be problematic or conflict with each other.
- Consider constructing similar scenarios or discuss in groups (with appropriate ground rules of mutual confidentiality and respect) professional dilemmas and areas relating to the competencies in the Person Specification.

The National Office for GP Recruitment does not recommend that you book commercial courses or purchase advice and guidance books specifically aimed at doctors undertaking the GP SAC. None of the GP assessors take part in or endorse any preparation courses or books. You may, however, treat such courses as an opportunity to: (1) refresh knowledge about professional responsibilities and ethical terminology, (2) network with colleagues and share experiences and (3) see 'where others are at' to reduce your own anxiety.

Box 7.1 Commercial courses and preparation for GP training assessments

---

On the day
- Be yourself and act naturally
- Be honest; assessors are not naive
- Listen and read carefully all instructions given on the day about the exercises
- Trust the process
- Evaluation to date says the process is fair, even from those who are not successful.

Sources of further information

Modernising Medical Careers: http://www.mmc.nhs.uk/

Postgraduate Medical Education and Training Board (PMETB): http://www.pmetb.org.uk/

National recruitment office for GP training: http://www.gprecruitment.org.uk/

8

Postgraduate exams

Key aims of this chapter

- Analyse the process of postgraduate exams
- Discuss thoughts on when to sit exams and tips on how to succeed at them
- Provide notes on specialty-specific exams.

Introduction

Postgraduate exams can be extremely daunting. Combining revision with your career is challenging and even the very best candidates find it hard to pass all parts at the first attempt. The key to understanding them is to realise that you are not actually expected to pass them all immediately and at the earliest attempt. Unlike finals at medical school, which are designed to exclude unsafe doctors and otherwise pass as many candidates as possible, these exams can sometimes seem to be designed to do the exact opposite.

Exams that result in entry to a Royal College are deliberately difficult. The written questions can be ambiguous and in the clinical sections the examiners may try to explicitly make you uncomfortable. The bar is set high enough so that only a certain percentage of applicants pass at each attempt. However, the majority of senior doctors who have passed such exams agree that although at the time they can seem extremely difficult, in hindsight they are no different to the many exams you will have taken during your time in medical school. Like those, they simply require hard work, determination even in the face of failure and, as always, a little luck.

Process of postgraduate exams

Specialty exams

Postgraduate exams are taken at set periods of time after graduation from medical school. They can often only be taken after the relevant clinical experience has been gained and this must be documented in the exam application. They consist of several parts spread out over a number of months or years. Typically the first parts of the exam concentrate on book knowledge and consist of multiple choice or extended matching questions. Each part can sometimes be taken independently of each other but they are usually sat in a step-wise manner with success at one part needed to guarantee progression to the next stage. The system is currently in flux but a general rule of thumb in hospital medicine is that success at a postgraduate exam is essential for the award of a certificate of completion of training (CCT) prior to becoming a consultant and is often also needed for progression beyond ST3.

Exams for specific specialties are often run through the relevant Royal Colleges, e.g. the MRCP is the exam undertaken by doctors wishing to specialise as physicians. Once general exams are passed there is often a need for further, more specialist exams, e.g. a doctor wishing to train as a clinical oncologist may have passed her MRCP during her core medical training jobs. After this she may decide to specialise in clinical oncology and will then have to pass her specialist exams to gain entry to the Royal College of Radiologists (who govern clinical or radiation oncology) before she is able to be appointed as a consultant.

Postgraduate exams set the bar for passing relatively high and the number of candidates who are successful at any given attempt can be as low as 20%. The examining body will usually decide on how many people they wish to pass at each attempt and this means that the pass mark is often not set in stone but can vary with the overall ability of the candidates sitting the exam.

Royal Colleges, Diplomas and Masters

The majority of postgraduate exams are held through the various Royal Colleges and success at them leads to acceptance as a Member of the Royal College. Alternative examinations that are needed for career progression may be awarded as Diplomas rather than as a Membership. These are not necessarily set through a Royal College, e.g. a number of clinicians wishing to pursue a career in infectious disease or tropical medicine may opt to study for a Diploma in Tropical Medicine and Hygiene, e.g. from the London School of Hygiene and Tropical Medicine. Diplomas are not always mandatory and are often taken in addition to Membership exams.

Another type of exam or postgraduate qualification is that of a Masters degree. This takes place through a university. It is often studied for part time or in your own time and may be directly relevant to your area of interest or indirectly useful, e.g. a Masters in Business Administration (MBA). It is essential to speak to senior doctors in your area of interest to find out what, if any, examinations or qualifications are recommended in addition to Royal College exams.

Exit exams

These exams are also known as knowledge-based assessments. Certain specialties such as surgery have used exit exams for a long period of time but for other fields the exams were borne out of Modernising Medical Careers. They were created as a joint collaboration between Specialist Societies (e.g. the British Thoracic Society in the case of respiratory medicine and the Federation of Royal Colleges of Physicians of the UK). The aim is to ensure that consultants or other specialist clinicians can practice medicine 'safely and competently'.

The advantage of such exams is that where previously a SpR would have been able to progress through the ranks with little or no formal assessment before being appointed as a consultant, they now have to demonstrate their suitability for the position. There is no current syllabus for any of the specialties other than the core competencies needed to practice, which will have been laid out as part of their training programme. The exams vary between specialties and may consist of written MCQ papers or oral assessments such as a viva. At the moment they are not always compulsory for old-style trainees (Specialist Registrars) but this may change.

Overseas exams and qualifications

UK-trained doctors who are considering practising overseas (even for a short period of time) should consider sitting any country-specific exams in conjunction with their own postgraduate exams. For example, the United States Medical Licensing Examination (USMLE) is needed to practice medicine in the USA. It consists of three sections called 'steps', which have similarities to existing examinations in the UK e.g. step 2 is an MCQ paper with clinical scenarios similar to that of part 2 of the Membership of the Royal Colleges of Physicians. It is important to review the syllabus carefully and to try to take the exams at the appropriate level of training. In addition, the score gained in the USMLEs is important, e.g. a higher score will be needed to practice in a competitive specialty or in a popular region of the country.

Graduates from countries outside of the European Economic Area will have to take the Professional and Linguistic Assessments Board (PLAB) exam to practice medicine in the UK. Again, it may be wise to sit the exam in conjunction with other exams, e.g. part 2 of the PLAB is an OSCE exam, which may be similar in format to an overseas examination.

MCQs, EMQs and SAQs

Multiple choice questions represent the bulk of the written parts of most postgraduate exams. They were traditionally a series of statements each of which could be true or false. After marking the answer sheet indicating whether you thought a statement was correct or not, the marks would be collated. In some cases 75% of questions would need to be answered correctly in order to pass and in other cases where negative marking was used (i.e. a wrong answer meant a mark of –1) the pass mark was closer to 50%. This style of question has largely been superseded by the *best of five format*.

In these MCQs each question begins with a stem that is usually a fact or a short clinical scenario. There are then five statements relating to the stem, one of which is the correct answer. Modern questions are usually designed so that a candidate who has prepared adequately will be able to immediately dismiss two of the statements as being incorrect. A third statement may be considered possible but the fourth and fifth statements could both be correct. The difficulty lies in deciding which of the two is the most correct.

If you do not immediately know the correct answer then the best method is to start by excluding the statements that are incorrect until you are finally left with a couple of statements from which to choose from. Often, there may be key words to help you come to an answer, e.g. a statement that reads 'You should **always** examine the neck first' is less likely to be correct than one that reads that 'You should **aim** to examine the neck first.' The best practice for MCQs is to complete as many questions as possible both in books, revision papers (if available) and on-line revision sites. Although you may not have repeats of questions in the actual exam there will be some similarity between stems and statements and by regularly practising them beforehand you will be in the correct frame of mind to tackle the questions.

Extended matching questions (EMQs) are a variation of MCQs with multiple stems and multiple statements. You may be asked to match the stems and statements that best fit together. The key to answering these is the same as with MCQs, i.e. practise as many as possible and if you are unsure of the correct answer then eliminate the possibilities until you are left with a smaller number of combinations from which to choose.

Short-answer questions (SAQs) are still used by some of the postgraduate medical bodies but they are almost always used in conjunction with MCQs. These are questions designed to allow the candidate to write a short and concise piece of information about a particular topic or scenario. The key to answering SAQs is to structure your answer carefully. It is wise to have a short introduction sentence as well as a brief conclusion. In some cases, higher marks can be scored by answering with bullet points or a series of statements, or even a diagram, rather than writing a paragraph of pure text. All examining boards will have examples of the best way in which to answer their own SAQs.

Objective structured clinical examinations

OSCEs make up the majority of clinical examinations both in medical school and for postgraduates. They are made up of a series of stations, each usually between 5- and 20-minutes long. Each station consists of a scenario such as a history-taking station, a clinical examination or a practical procedure. An examiner marks the candidate and the overall scores are collated to determine whether the candidate has passed or failed. The pass mark, like many other parts of postgraduate examinations, is fluid and changes depending on the strength or weaknesses of other candidates who sit the exam at the same time.

The conventional wisdom with OSCEs is that practise makes perfect. Often, the stations can be predicted beforehand and it is important to have worked out how the scenario will unfold, e.g. in the Membership of the Royal Colleges of Physicians OSCE the clinical examination stations are divided up by system. The vast majority of cardiovascular examination stations will fall into four or five scenarios and it is important to have thought these through and be prepared for any questions that the examiner may ask afterwards.

The nature of the examination means that it has to occur at several sites over a period of time. Whilst most of the patients and scenarios differ between exams there is the potential for repetition, meaning that candidates who sit the examination towards the end of the period may have an advantage if they have spoken to colleagues who have already sat the exam.

Clinical long cases

These are being phased out from the current round of postgraduate examinations. They were traditionally used in several formats depending on the length of time spend with a patient. Long cases would typically range from 20–30 minutes and allow a candidate to spend that time with a patient to take a full history and perform an appropriate examination. They would then be asked questions before being taken back to the patient to demonstrate any appropriate physical signs.

Short cases are similar to OSCEs in that a pair of examiners take a candidate on a circuit of several patients each lasting only a few minutes. They would then be asked to examine specific systems or point out clinical signs before answering a set number of questions.

Thoughts on when to sit exams and tips on how to succeed at them

When to take postgraduate examinations

The conventional wisdom is that there is no good time to take postgraduate exams. The first few years after graduating from medical school can be both exciting and demanding. There is much to learn about the process of being a doctor and exams are not at the forefront of most people's minds. Indeed, it may be a few years before a final choice of career is chosen. This is a valid point to bear in mind and you might want to experience a few different specialties before making up your mind about long-term career goals. However, for clinicians who know the area in which they want to specialise, the best advice is to take the exams at the earliest possible opportunity and often this is in the first foundation year.

There are a number of reasons for this attitude. Medical students cram a lot into their university exams and much of that information can form a solid base from which to study for postgraduate exams. The sooner these are taken, the more likely it is that you will be able to use the information learned from medical school. In addition, the keenest and most hard working of colleagues will aim to sit exams as soon as possible. Even if you are not in that category you could benefit hugely from revising with others who are sitting the exams at the same time as you.

Most students graduate with student loans and a somewhat limited first income but the majority of this is often disposable since many will not yet have bought a home or started a family. Exams cost a great deal of money from books to online question sites, revision courses, and the actual exams themselves, which can cost a remarkable amount of money. Failing them means that you will have to pay again and it may be wiser to get them out of the way before your income is spent on a mortgage, a wedding or child support payments.

There is also the advantage to your future career of sitting exams early. Many of your colleagues may have waited until they felt they were clinically experienced to do so. Most senior doctors have realised that the process of revising for postgraduate exams is a teaching method in itself and there is no reason to delay them. By passing part or all of an exam it will give you a strong footing when applying for a training position as it will let a shortlisting panel know that you were determined and enthusiastic about their specialty from the beginning. Your colleagues who have not yet sat any exams will be unable to demonstrate.

Revision courses

Each part of a postgraduate exam can attract a number of revision courses. These are often very expensive and it can be hard to try to distinguish the better ones from the rest of the crowd. The key task here is to speak to senior doctors within the specialty. Find out which courses they attended and what they thought of them and then search online for user comments about the courses. Often the most expensive courses with the glossiest advertisements are not the best ones.

Revision courses can be in large rooms if lecturers are going over a number of topics for a written exam and they can take up several weekends or an entire week of evening lectures. These occur in the larger cities, with London having the greatest selection of courses and dates. Smaller group teaching sessions will be available for clinical exams but these are much more expensive as they require payment to more tutors as well as to volunteer patients.

A number of courses are available online and these include databases of MCQs and EMQs as well as video tutorials looking at clinical scenarios. The advantage of these is that they are significantly cheaper than real revision courses and you can look at them whenever you have a free moment. In the case of MCQs you are usually able to organise the questions into sections, attempt only those that you have not done before and compare your scores online with other candidates.

In all cases it is usually helpful to attend one or more revision course, particularly when sitting the clinical parts of exams. These are best done in conjunction with colleagues so that you can compare notes after the session and provide each other with support during later revision sessions. Although they may seem expensive, they will probably increase your chances of passing and the costs will be minimal compared to those of repeat examination fees and time spent revising the same topics a second time. Exam fees, books and payments for revision courses are tax deductible for those who fill in a yearly tax return. However, it is important to note that revision courses are not essential and self-motivated hard-working junior doctors will be able to pass without them.

Personalised revision notes

Revision for exams in medical school are often centred on lecture notes. There are no universally defined notes for postgraduate exams and so it is important to make your own personalised set of notes based on the available sources. Each specialty will have a limited number (often just one) of textbooks that the majority of candidates revise from and these should form the basis of your own revision notes.

Added to these should be notes made from revision courses, online notes and points made from group study sessions. If using MCQ question books then make sure you annotate them to help you remember essential points. Try and speak to senior colleagues who have sat the exams already as they may be willing to share their own notes and revision experiences with you.

Study with others

This may be a technique learnt from medical school but if not then it is essential that you begin now. Postgraduate exams are significantly harder than those at university and finding a group of colleagues to revise with will help increase your chances of passing. This may be simply going over MCQs with another junior doctor in the mess or talking through a series of topics after a ward round.

In the case of clinical examinations this becomes even more important. You will learn little by practising examination of a patient's knee joint by

A number of hospitals and GP training schemes are cutting back on study leave both in terms of the amount of days that you are entitled to as well as the financial assistance given but are still obliged to provide a minimum number of days and money to doctors in training (FY1 doctors and those not in recognised training programmes are currently not entitled to any study leave). It is important for clinicians who are entitled to make the most use of anything that is available. This may mean swapping on-call commitments or shift work and these should be sorted out well in advance of the necessary time.

Leave can be taken to attend exam revision courses, to sit the exams or for private study. In the latter case, all such leave should be saved up for the week leading up to the exam so that you give yourself the best possible opportunity of passing. Study leave can also be given for attendance at professional development courses and scientific meetings but unless you are confident about your revision, all leave should be saved for activities related to exams. Once you pass your exams there will be ample opportunity to travel to conferences and meetings.

Box 8.1 Study leave entitlement

yourself. Instead, find a number of colleagues to work with. Set up a teaching rota for the weeks leading up to the exams and cajole some senior doctors into joining this rota. Have a list of patients in hospital with good clinical stories or signs and ask someone to watch you and your colleagues interact with the patient as if it were a real exam. Expect to be asked questions and be marked critically and then discuss the cases with each other at a later date. By working together you will markedly increase your chances of passing an exam.

How to balance revision with the rest of your life

Unlike medical school, where you can simply study for your exams, the difficulty with postgraduate exams is that you have to sit them whilst working in a demanding career. As time passes you have to incorporate the ever-increasing complexity of your personal life into this and the ability to focus on exams will become harder. There are methods of achieving a good work–life balance whilst still concentrating on your exams.

The best thing to do is to try and do as much work at work. This may seem straightforward but it is vital that you use all opportunities that are given to you during your normal working hours rather than revising at home.

There are often periods of quiet between clinics, after a ward round or when an on-call is under control and there are no patients to be seen. If you are revising for exams then it is essential that you have revision material available at all times. This may be in the form of a pocket book, a few pages of handwritten notes or access to an online question database that you can surf at 3am when on a restful night shift. By shifting the focus of exams away from your home life and into work you will be able to achieve a better balance.

Notes on specialty-specific exams

The notes below are details for a number of the most common postgraduate examinations within the UK. They do not cover all specialties. The details are correct at the current time but all examination formats are likely to change over time and up-to-date details can be found on the websites of the relevant exam bodies.

Specialty: Medicine
Body: Royal College of Physicians
Website: http:// www.mrcpuk.org
Exam format: Doctors must have had at least 12 months' experience in medical employment, i.e. have completed FY1 or equivalent before applying and sitting the exam, and they must have discussed their proposed application with their educational supervisor.

The exam consists of three parts. Part 1 can be taken an unlimited number of times. It consists of two 3-hour papers each with 100 MCQs in one from five (best of five) format. They cover a wide range of subjects including statistics, biochemistry and physiology as well as the system-based sciences such as cardiology or respiratory medicine. These questions are designed to test a candidate's knowledge and understanding of the clinical sciences relevant to medical practice.

Part 2 written will test your ability to apply clinical understanding and make clinical judgements. As well as medical questions there are some on adolescent medicine and psychiatry. The format is the same as Part 1 with two 3-hour papers each and 100 MCQs in one from five (best of five) format.

PACES is aimed to demonstrate in a clinical setting, the knowledge, skills and attitudes appropriate for a physician. The exam consists of an OSCE scenario with stations on physical examination, identifying physical signs, clinical communication, differential diagnosis, clinical judgement, managing patients' concerns and maintaining patients' welfare.

Specialty: Surgery
Body: Royal College of Surgeons
Website: http://www.intercollegiatemrcs.org.uk
Exam format: The exam format has recently changed. Prior to 2008 it was offered in three parts but for all candidates who have not yet started on the old system there will be a new method of examination consisting of just two parts.

Part 1 consists of two 2-hour MCQ papers, the first of which concerns applied basic sciences, which covers subjects including physiology, anatomy and pathology. The second MCQ paper concerns principles of surgery in general and covers subjects including perioperative care, postoperative management, critical care issues, microbiology and surgical technique and technology.

Part 2 is OSCE scenario with stations covering anatomy and surgical pathology, surgical skills and patient safety, communication skills, applied surgical science and critical care and clinical skills in history taking and physical examination. The timing of the exams is not restricted and they can be taken at any stage of surgical training.

Specialty: General practice
Body: Royal College of General Pracitioners
Website: http://www.rcgp.org.uk
Exam format: The exam format has recently changed and is now an integrated assessment programme that includes three components. Each part is independent of the other but all must be attained in order for the Membership to be conferred.

The workplace-based assessment consists of 12 areas of professional competence against which evidence is gathered using designated and validated tools. These include a patient satisfaction questionnaire, a direct observation of procedural skills and a clinical evaluation exercise. The assessment is carried out during the 3 years of GP training placements.

The clinical skills assessment occurs in the form of an OSCE with a number of patient consultations to assess problem-solving skills, attitude and primary care management. There will also be the opportunity to assess physical examination skills and the appropriate use of diagnostic equipment.

The applied knowledge test is a written examination that is taken on a computer and consists of a 3-hour MCQ exam with 200 questions. The topics cover clinical medicine (80% of questions), critical appraisal and evidence-based clinical practice (10%) and health informatics and administrative issues (10%).

Specialty: Psychiatry
Body: Royal College of General Psychiatrists
Website: http://www.rcpsych.ac.uk
Exam format: There are three written papers, each 3 hours in duration and consisting of 200 questions, which are either in the MCQ best of five format or presented as EMQs. The topics covered include history and mental state examination, cognitive assessment, prevention of psychiatric disorders and dynamic psychopathology.

The clinical assessment of skills and competencies (CASC) part of the exam is in the format of an OSCE. The syllabus for this part of the exam covers general adult psychiatry, old age psychiatry, learning disability, psychotherapy and forensic psychiatry.

Specialty: Paediatrics
Body: Royal College of Paediatricians
Website: http://www.rcpch.ac.uk
Exam format: The exam is taken during the period of basic specialist training and consists of three parts. Part 1 consists of two papers. The first paper focuses on the areas of child health that are relevant to those who will be working with children in their medical careers and is not just applicable to paediatricians. The second paper assesses complex paediatric problem-solving skills and the scientific knowledge underpinning paediatrics. Both papers consist of extended matching questions, multiple true/false questions and best of five MCQs.

Part 2 consists of two papers with MCQs and best of five questions. The questions revolve around data interpretation, photographic material and clinical scenarios. The clinical examination follows a traditional OSCE format and assesses areas including child development, communication skills, history taking, management planning, recognition and diagnosis of clinical signs and symptoms, and physical examination skills.

Specialty: Anaesthetics

Body: Royal College of Anaesthetists

Website: http://www.rcoa.ac.uk

Exam format: The Fellowship of the Royal College of Anaesthetists (FRCA) is divided into two parts. Part 1 (the Primary) is taken during the period of specialist training. The Primary consists of two sections. The first section is a multiple choice paper consisting of 90 true/false questions with no negative marking. Topics covered include pharmacology, physiology, biochemistry, physics, clinical measurement and data interpretation. The second part of the Primary consist of an 18-station OSCE covering topics including resuscitation, technical skills, anatomy, history taking, physical examination, communication skills, anaesthetic equipment and monitoring equipment as well as a 1-hour viva (called a structured oral examination), which covers physiology, biochemistry and clinical incidents.

Part 2 (Final) also comprises of two sections. The first section involves a 90-question MCQ exam covering medicine and surgery, anaesthesia and pain management, applied basic sciences, clinical measurement and intensive therapy as well as a 3-hour short-answer question on the principles and practices of clinical anaesthesia. The second section can only be taken once you have passed the first section of the Final FRCA and consists of two vivas covering clinical anaesthesia and clinical science.

Specialty: Radiology

Body: Royal College of Radiologists

Website: http://www.rcr.ac.uk

Exam format: The exam is taken during the period of specialist training and consists of two parts. Part 1 of the FRCR examination comprises two modules in physics and radiological anatomy. The physics sections comprise of a 2-hour true/false-style MCQ examination with no negative marking. The anatomy part lasts for 75 minutes and comprises 20 cases/images, with five questions about each case. Each candidate is assigned to a computer workstation for the duration of the exam.

The second part of the FRCR can only be taken after successful completion of the first part. Part A comprises of six separate single best answer MCQ papers covering imaging of a number of areas including cardiothoracic and vascular, musculoskeletal and trauma, gastrointestinal (including liver, biliary, pancreas and spleen, genitourinary, adrenal, obstetrics and gynaecology and breast, paediatric, central nervous, and head and neck (including spine, eyes, ENT, salivary glands and dental). Part B consists of a reporting session, a rapid reporting session and two oral examinations.

Specialty: Clinical oncology
Body: Royal College of Radiologists
Website: http://www.rcr.ac.uk
Exam format: The Royal College of Radiology is the body responsible for postgraduate examinations in clinical oncology. The examination is divided into two parts. The first part consists of four MCQ (single best answer) papers covering cancer biology and radiobiology, clinical pharmacology, physics and medical statistics.

Part 2 consists of three sections. The first involves two MCQ (single best answer) papers each comprising of 120 questions covering all aspects of clinical oncology and radiotherapy planning. The second part comprises a 40-minute OSCE involving patient examination and management as well as interpretation of data and investigations. The final part consists of a 40-minute viva from two examiners covering all aspects of the specialty.

Specialty: Obstetrics and gynaecology
Body: Royal College of Obstetrics and Gynaecology
Website: http://www.rcog.org.uk
Exam format: The exam is taken during the period of specialist training and consists of two parts. Part 1 consists of two papers. Both papers consist of EMQs as well as standard MCQs with true/false stems. The questions cover topics including IT, core surgical care, antenatal care, postoperative care, maternal medicine, surgical procedures, management of delivery, subfertility, oncology and sexual and reproductive health.

Part 2 consist of two parts. The first part is a written examination with questions covering all aspects of the specialty and is examined using a mixture of EMQs, MCQs and SAQs. The second part is in an OSCE format and covers topics which include describing an operation in detail, history taking, clinical prioritisation, surgical skills, audit and critical appraisal.

Specialty: Pathology
Body: Royal College of Pathology
Website: http://www.rcpath.org
Exam format: The Royal College of Pathology is the postgraduate body responsible for administering postgraduate examinations in

a number of fields. The examinations vary for the type of specialty but include specialties as diverse as clinical biochemistry, clinical embryology, clinical cytogenetics, clinical molecular genetics, haematology, histopathology, immunology, medical microbiology, neuropathology, oral pathology, toxicology, veterinary clinical pathology, and virology.

Sources of further information

Postgraduate Medical Education and Training Board (PMETB): http://www.pmetb.org.uk

The Joint College of Physicians Training Board: http://www.jrcptb.org.uk

Professional Linguistics and Assessment Board exams (PLAB): http://www.gmc-uk. org/doctors/plab.asp

United States Medical Licensing Examination (USMLE): http://www.usmle.org

9

Audit

Key aims of this chapter

- Detail the background to audits and the discuss the difference types of audit used in clinical medicine
- Describe the audit process in detail
- Discuss tips on how to become involved with audit and how to choose audits that are novel, important and useful to further your career.

Introduction

On paper, an audit can be deceptively easy to plan and carry out. You need to decide on an important issue and investigate whether or not things are being carried out to the highest standard of practice. For example, a chest physician may want to see if her department is following the hospital's local policy on carrying out a bronchoscopy on all patients with suspected lung cancer within 10 days. She may decide to do this by looking at all patient notes over a period of 3 months and working out how long it took for them to have the procedure and then reporting back to the department. But is this the best way of doing it?

Why has she chosen to look back over 3 months rather than 6 months? Will she look at her own patients or those from the whole department and should she compare these to those from a nearby hospital within the same Primary Care Trust (PCT)? Are her hospital's guidelines the same as those from the British Thoracic Society? If not, why are they different and should she use ones from a national society instead? Does the British Thoracic Society have the best guidance?

Does she take into account the route of referral to the bronchoscopy suite, for example, should patients from the chest clinic be treated differently to those referred as inpatients from other teams? If the hospital is not meeting their own guidelines, then would interventions at the point of seeing the patient be more beneficial than those interventions made from the bronchoscopy suite itself?

Audit is often a stand-alone question on a job application form and so merely being involved with a clinical audit can no longer be used to differentiate between candidates at interview. The level of involvement, thought processes behind the audit and the measures put in place to improve the outcome will be crucial in selecting those who have gone the extra mile and produced a good rather than a standard audit.

Definition of audit

There are many recognised definitions of an audit and they differ slightly depending on the exact area that is being audited. A simple and widely used definition is that an audit is the 'evaluation of a process, organisation, product or person that is carried out in a systematic manner, resulting in the identification of interventions that can be used to improve the original process'. The NHS Executive describes a clinical audit as "the systematic analysis of the quality of healthcare, including the procedures used for diagnosis, treatment and care, the use of resources and the resulting outcome and quality of life for the patient".

NICE gives a more formal definition of a clinical audit as being "a quality improvement process that seeks to improve patient care and outcomes through systematic review of care against explicit criteria and the implementation of change. Aspects of the structure, processes, and outcomes of care are selected and systematically evaluated against explicit criteria. Where indicated, changes are implemented at an individual, team, or service level and further monitoring is used to confirm improvement in healthcare delivery".

Although definitions may vary, the end product of all audits is not a fixed point. Instead, any changes as a result of interventions will have to be re-evaluated to see if they have indeed resulted in an improvement. In this manner, the audit cycle continues and it is important that all audits have a mechanism for this continuation and re-evaluation.

Audits, assessments and investigations

An audit is an independent evaluation, often of a process. The person carrying out the audit can be part of the system but the auditing itself is independent to the process. By comparison, an assessment is often a two-way process with both the assessor and the assessee contributing to the final report. This level of consultation is not seen in an audit that usually starts with a fixed objective and there is no feedback until the process is complete.

Unlike an audit, an assessment ends with a report and whilst there may be suggestions to improve performance, these do not necessarily have to be implemented or re-assessed. An investigation is also different to an audit in that it ends with a report that apportions blame or praise on a process. There is no direct mechanism for intervention and further investigations.

History of audits

Financial audits

The financial world uses audits to a far greater degree than in medicine and understanding a financial audit may help explain why good audits can be important and have real-world consequences in any setting. Cases such as the Enron scandal in the USA showed that inaccurate auditing of financial statements, amongst other transgressions, helped to bankrupt the multibillion dollar energy company.

Financial audits have occurred for centuries and in the UK the position of Auditor of the Exchequer was first mentioned in 1314. In 1866 the Exchequer and Audit Departments Act was set up by the then Chancellor of the Exchequer and asked all Government departments to provide accurate audited accounts.

Financial audits are however different to clinical audits in that after the evaluation of finances, there is no continuation of the cycle. Instead, an audit report is produced, which provides an expert opinion on whether financial statements from an organisation are indeed accurate.

Medical audits

Perhaps the most famous early example of a clinical audit is that of Florence Nightingale, who used a methodical approach to dramatically reduce mortality amongst injured soldiers in the Crimean War in the middle of the nineteenth century. After noticing a poor level of basic hygiene on the wards, she introduced a new regimen involving basic sanitation and postoperative care.

Her mathematical background allowed her to calculate the impact of these changes on mortality and over a 4-month period the mortality rate dropped by one-third from 60% to 40%. A re-evaluation of the audit process by her and the introduction of fresh fruit and clean water enabled a further dramatic reduction to just 2% within a further few months.

Examples of major current UK national clinical audits include evaluations of the quality and delivery of care for children and young people with suspected and diagnosed epilepsies, prescribing practice for treatment-resistant schizophrenia and a quality improvement programme for the national pain database.

People involved with audit

For each individual audit, a lead auditor takes a role in preparing the background to the audit, designing the audit itself, carrying it out, and analysing the data. The clinical lead may be internal, e.g. a junior doctor within a surgical team evaluating postoperative infection rates within his own general surgical team or they may be external, e.g. an ophthalmic surgeon brought in by the general surgeons to provide a more independent audit. The clinical lead will also be involved with suggestions for interventions to improve the process and they will be responsible for the presentation of the audit's findings to the interested parties.

A second lead auditor is needed to repeat the audit after any suggested interventions have occurred to see whether or not they have resulted in improvements to the process. This person may be the original clinician but in many instances it is preferable to have the re-evaluation carried out by a second individual to reduce bias. In cases of audits being carried out by junior members of the team, the time factor between audits means that for practical purposes it is often a new team member who carries out the second audit.

Many hospital departments have committees to oversee clinical audits. This may consist of a board of senior doctors or may be open to all members of a particular department. They will meet on an infrequent but regular basis to review all ongoing audits in their specialty and propose new audits as well as close the loop on older audits that have occurred in the past.

Depending on the type of clinical audit, the lead auditor and people interested in the audit may be medical staff, nursing staff, those from allied professions or members of management. In some cases, the audit can transgress across multidisciplinary fields and have far-reaching consequences outside of that originally intended by the lead auditor, e.g. an audit evaluating waiting times for hip replacement surgery in a hospital may be carried out by an FY1 doctor in orthopaedic surgery with help from the appropriate consultant.

Presentation of the audit's findings may take place to: (1) orthopaedic surgeons who wish to reduce their waiting times, (2) vascular surgeons who want to see if they can learn anything from the processes used, (3) occupational therapists who want to see if they can introduce walking aids to pre-operative patients earlier than at present and to (4) senior hospital managers who want to meet national targets to cut waiting times and so earn the hospital a financial bonus which can be used to buy modern ventilator equipment for the neonatal intensive care unit.

Clinical governance

The ever-changing face of modern medicine, particularly within the UK's NHS means that a number of different definitions of topics associated with audit have been proposed in recent years. The majority have not been universally accepted, primarily due to the increasing complexity of definitions. However, one area in which there has been much agreement is with the use of the term 'clinical governance'.

In recent years, clinical governance has been used as an umbrella term to describe a number of different processes that contribute towards improving patient care. The UK Department of Health defines clinical governance as "the system through which NHS organisations are accountable for continuously improving the quality of their services and safeguarding high standards of care, by creating an environment in which clinical excellence will flourish".

Types of audit

There are several ways of classifying the different types of audit. One method would be to classify them as clinical and non-clinical.

Clinical governance covers seven processes that are sometimes called the 'seven pillars of governance'. These processes have been altered over time to take into account changing trends within the NHS but have a core set of criteria:

1. Clinical audit as explained in this chapter
2. Service user, carer and public involvement, which takes into account the increased need of the NHS to be open to users with particular regard to areas of difficulty such as rationing of care and waiting lists
3. Risk management, which can cover clinical or managerial risk
4. Research and development, which covers basic, translational and clinical research
5. Education and training of students, doctors and other health professionals
6. Clinical effectiveness of specific treatments, interventions and therapies
7. Clinical information with particular regard to access of up-to-date and relevant information by healthcare professionals

Box 9.1 Seven pillars of clinical audit

Clinical audits

These would evaluate specific processes that have direct impact on patient care, e.g. rates of post-procedural bleeding after gastric biopsy or the number of patients on a cardiac ward that are put on beta-blocker medication post myocardial infarction.

Non-clinical audits

These are audits that do not have a direct impact on patient care but nonetheless have a bearing on the management of patients in general, e.g. an evaluation of the length of time taken to carry out a cataract operation from first referral to a specialist. Other examples of non-clinical audits in medicine include those that are management or laboratory based.

Clinical audits can be vastly different in scope and outcome depending on the process, target audience and motivation of the lead auditor. They can be further divided up depending on exactly what is being evaluated. The different forms can be applied across the board in the different clinical specialties and are not always mutually exclusive of one another.

1. Standards-based audit

This defines what is historically thought of as a straightforward clinical audit. A particular process or system is investigated to see if the current standards are being met. Data is collected and analysed to see whether this is the case. If not, the results of the audit are presented to the interested parties and interventions suggested to improve the outcome.

An example of this is that of an FY2 trainee in renal medicine in a large teaching hospital who wonders whether all of the patients who need emergency dialysis are receiving it by the appropriate time. The in-house hospital protocol states that all patients who are admitted with acute renal failure and who are appropriate for intervention should have emergency dialysis started within 6 hours.

The trainee and consultant discuss this and they decide that it would be a worthwhile audit to carry out. In order not to miss any patients, he analyses both the dialysis ward's notes and those of all emergency admissions to the hospital over a 6-month period. This is made easier by the fact that all emergency admissions are coded on the electronic case records, making the search relatively straightforward. He identifies a number of patients and finds that only half of the admissions that need dialysis are receiving it within 6 hours but almost all are receiving it within 12 hours.

The trainee presents these findings to the entire renal team, which consists of doctors, ward nurses and community nurses as well as to a number of the acute and emergency physicians. The trainee's ideas for intervention to improve the standard of care include a red flag attached to the electronic notes of all emergency admissions with acute renal failure, the notification of one of the renal consultants during working hours of all acute admissions and the notification of the nurse in charge of the renal ward at night and at the weekend by the admitting doctor to speed things up. Some of these suggestions are implemented over a 3-month period and it is agreed that the audit is to be carried out again following this.

2. Senior review audit

This type of clinical audit is usually carried out on an infrequent but regular basis by a group of senior clinicians. They may review processes or systems or individual medical cases with a view to evaluate the standards of care in each case. They will make recommendations and evaluate the effectiveness of these at a future meeting. Unlike a standards-based audit, there is no formal mechanism for re-evaluation.

An example of this type of audit is the 'morbidity and mortality' meetings carried out in some hospitals. The audits are usually led by senior surgeons with much of their team in attendance. Figures for overall mortality and morbidity for specific teams and specific conditions are evaluated and a number of clinical cases are discussed with a view to see if those patients received the best standard of care. Areas in which interventions would have improved the outcome are discussed in detail and noted for the future.

3. Critical incident audit

This type of audit is similar to the senior review audit in that it is often carried out by senior members of the team. It differs in that rather than looking at a process or standard, individual critical incidents are examined over a period of time. The incidents are discussed by the entire multidisciplinary team with a view to looking for trends or similarities between incidents. Ideas for interventions are discussed and noted for the future to prevent such incidents.

An example of this type of audit is of a regular meeting of a psychiatric department examining all critical incidents involving staff and patient safety over a period of time. The audit involves doctors, specialist nurses and receptionists from the outpatient department and from the ward. A trend is noted with an increased number of verbal threats against receptionists in the outpatient department and it is noted that this may be due to the clinics running much later in previous months and the lack of communication of this to patients. It is decided that an appropriate intervention would be to inform patients on arrival of the estimated waiting time past their expected appointment to see if this lowers the number of critical incidents in this area.

4. Patient-centred audit

This type of audit involves patients rather than clinicians and aims to examine the patients' attitudes to the care they have received. It may be systematic in that it is carried out over a period of time for a set number of patients and that all views are collated for discussion by the clinical team.

An example of this type of audit is of a neonatal consultant wondering whether the parents of newborn babies feel adequately involved in their care on the neonatal intensive care unit. He gives questionnaires to 30 randomly selected parents over a 4-month period and asks them to

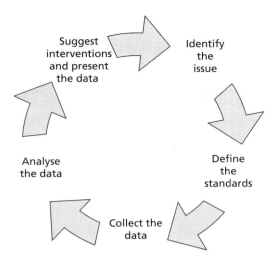

Figure 9.1 The audit cycle

score a number of specific statements regarding visiting times, interactions with nurses and explanations of conditions by the doctors. The results are collated and analysed before being discussed with the entire department. There is a general consensus by parents that they would like more information on a daily basis by the visiting consultants. The extra time needed for this is factored into the existing ward rounds and agreed by all the clinicians.

Audit cycle

The audit cycle encompasses a number of steps that need to be completed in order for the audit to succeed:

Step 1 – Identify issue to be evaluated

Choosing an issue

The lead auditor should identify a particular issue of concern to be evaluated. This is often an issue within their area of expertise such as their clinical field, area of management or even area within the hospital, e.g. an outpatient co-ordinator may wish to audit waiting list times within her outpatient department across all the specialties.

Patient care

In addition to choosing an issue that is of interest to the lead auditor, the topic should be one that has bearing on patient care. This issue may have a direct bearing on patient care, e.g. when evaluating postoperative complications or an indirect bearing, e.g. the evaluation of patient information for those undergoing a particular procedure. The topic could be of importance to a large number of patients or, if the issue is important enough, it may only be applicable to a small number of patients, e.g. the auditing of chemotherapy drug usage for a rare type of cancer.

Problem issues

At its heart, the issue should be associated with a particular problem. The audit of a system or process that is generally thought to be working well is unhelpful, unless the lead auditor believes that the current conceptual standards are incorrect. The problem should be well defined, e.g. when evaluating the prophylaxis of thromboembolisms on a medical ward the problem should be seen as whether or not all patients are given thromboembolism prophylaxis in the form of stockings or low-molecular-weight heparin.

Areas of concern

A successful audit demands the interest of the lead auditor and it is best to get opinions from colleagues, patients and hospital management. There may be a particular area that has been a problem for a period of time and there may already be initial evaluation into that area that could be provided as a useful background to begin an audit, e.g. a GP partner may have noticed that she has had a problem with diabetic patients not being followed up regularly. She may already have some data on the numbers of patients who have missed their routine appointments and this would be a good starting place for a new GP trainee to begin. In addition, the hospital management or PCT may have particular problem areas that they wish audited.

Potential for improvement

The issue at heart should have room for substantial and real improvement otherwise the identification of problems through the audit will have no way of intervening to change things in the future, e.g. it may be well known that a particular hospital is having difficulty getting inpatients seen by the consultant neurologists who have to share their time amongst three different hospitals. An audit showing this may be useful in terms of backing up the argument to get better input but if the hospital management already know this and have explained that there will be no funding for further neurology input until the next financial year, then a small audit evaluating ten patients over a 6-month period may in itself be unhelpful.

Step 2 – Define the standards

Once the issue to be evaluated has been identified, a standard has to be decided upon. This standard forms the benchmark for the audit and is the marker for which all the data that is collected should be measured against.

Existing standard

The likely scenario is that the standard used is already in place. For example, an ST3 doctor in gastroenterology may decide to investigate the time taken for a patient with bleeding oesophageal varices to have an endoscopy as they may be concerned that some patients have to wait too long. There may be an existing 'internal standard' put in place from the hospital itself that states that all appropriate patients should have a therapeutic endoscopy within 4 hours. The standard may be initiated by his consultant, who would like all patients coming in as an emergency under her team to have an endoscopy within 3 hours. However, there may be an 'external standard' that has been put in place from a particular organisation, e.g. the British Society of Gastroenterology.

New standards

It may be the case that although a particular process or system has been decided upon, there is no existing standard in place. This may be because it simply hasn't been agreed upon before or it may be that it is a relatively new problem and so no standards have been created, e.g. a psychiatry FY1 trainee wonders whether other trainees are consulting online databases before prescribing drugs to patients. He discusses this with his consultant, who points out that the hospital has an up-to-date subscription to the latest national drug formulary and that all doctors should be consulting this to look for drug reactions and interactions before prescribing any new medication. There are no existing internal or external standards so the FY1 trainee and the consultant agree a new standard stating that at least 80% of all new prescriptions should have been evaluated using the online drug formulary prior to prescription.

Step 3 – Collect the data

Measurement against the standard

The standard chosen for the audit will be the benchmark against which the data is collected. There may be multiple standards but in many cases there is only one main standard that the data will be evaluated against, e.g. the standard for a basic biochemistry result being available on a hospital computer may have been defined as within 2 hours of sending off the sample during working hours. This is the main standard to which the data collected will be evaluated but there may be other standards used in addition, e.g. the time allowed to process samples may be longer at night or on weekends.

Choosing a frame of reference

These are the parameters for data collection. It may be a time reference, e.g. the evaluation of all patient notes from a 3-month period or it may be a numerical reference, e.g. the auditing of patients' attitudes from the past 50 patients to attend a genetics outpatient appointment. If previous audits into the same issue are available, this frame of reference should be checked against them.

Accurate data collection

It is important for the integrity of the audit that all data is collected as accurately as possible. This means that the data collection methods should be standardised, e.g. it may be that only one individual is responsible for data collection or if there are multiple auditors, there is a clear consensus on how the data is collected. The lead auditor should try hard to make sure that no data is missing, e.g. if notes are unavailable for the audit from a number of important patients then all effort should be made to find them.

Step 4 – Analyse the data

Evalation of data versus standards

The collated data needs to be analysed against the chosen standard. This may be straightforward and can take place without any further investigation, e.g. when looking to see if patients are seen in an outpatient clinic within a specific number of weeks from initial referral the data may simply state the percentage of patients that were. In other instances the data may require further analysis to see if the standards are met, e.g. an audit looking into times taken for histological diagnoses to be made from suspected lung cancer biopsies may require the times recorded to take into account further information such as methods of transportation of samples to the laboratory and annual leave of the reviewing histopathologists.

Analysis of why data does not meet standards

In cases where the analysed data does not meet the expected standard a further investigation needs to be undertaken to see if there are any commonalities within the data. For example, it may be that 20% of all lymph node biopsies are not being reported within the standard of 5 days. Within that 20%, a greater proportion may have been taken by surgical consultant A than consultant B. This operator difference may be the answer to why the standards are not being met, e.g. consultant A operates on a Friday and the intervening weekend causes a delay in reporting.

Step 5 – Suggested interventions for improvement and presentation of data

Suggestions for improvement

Once the data has been fully analysed and in some cases found not to meet the standard, there should be suggestions for improvement. For example, the audit may have evaluated the number of patients with COPD given smoking cessation advice in a general practice. The findings may be that only 70% of new diagnoses were being given advice over a 3-month period whereas the internal standard decided upon by the practice was 100%. The suggested interventions to improve the figures may include patient leaflets to be placed directly in notes by receptionist staff prior to consultations and a standard proforma for use by doctors when seeing COPD patients for the first time that includes a section on smoking cessation advice.

Presentation of data

The audit should be presented to all interested parties. This would include clinicians, nurses, allied health professionals and managers from within the relevant department. It may also include members from outside the department who may have an interest in the findings. The audit should be presented methodically with an explanation of the background to the issue, the reason for choosing the specific standards, how the data was collected and analysed, and a summary of the findings.

Points of action

Where standards are found not to be met, a series of interventions should be discussed that could be used to improve standards. These may have been discussed with senior members of staff prior to the presentation or they may be simply recorded as issues that will allow action points to be made during the presentation. The action should be recorded as part of the audit cycle and named individuals should be tasked with carrying them out over a set time period.

Step 6 – Repeat the audit

In order to close the audit loop, the audit should be carried out again after an agreed period of time. This will allow for any of the interventions to have occurred. The data collection and analysis should be exactly as before and be carried out by the same individuals or by other team members who have been instructed on exactly how to proceed. Once this is done, the data should be presented again.

If the standards have been improved to a satisfactory degree it may be deemed that the audit is over and that the loop has been closed. However if the improvement is not found, a new set of interventions may have to be agreed upon and then carried out before a further re-audit. Finally, it may be decided that the original standards were set too high and these may have to be lowered in order to complete the audit. Alternatively, it may be decided that for a particular case the standards of care are not being met and a more radical overhaul of the system is needed.

How to make the most of your audit and then sell it to an interview committee

Find existing audits

Whilst it is always preferable to initiate an audit yourself, a fast and simple way to get into the audit cycle is to find an existing audit and volunteer to continue it. The majority of clinical audits undertaken by junior doctors only exist in one cycle. Whilst they are always intended to be continued, this is often not the case due to not enough time, lack of initiative and the lead auditor moving out of the department. Most clinical teams will have audits in place that have been forgotten about. Discuss these with the clinicians in charge. In some cases the audits may be of low quality and in others they may represent data that is now of little interest. Find those audits that are relatively current, useful and easy to continue in your current setting.

Once you have chosen the audit, it is important to contact the lead auditor to both get their permission to continue the audit as well as to get inside tips on how to conduct it. Although there should be a written protocol for data collection and analysis, it is useful to speak to someone to see if there are any minor changes to the protocols and find out what difficulties they had in collecting and analysing the data.

At the presentation stage it is important to see if any of the suggested interventions have improved the outcome. If they have, the audit loop can be closed. If not, further suggestions to improve the outcome should be suggested and implemented.

Find existing data

Although previous high-quality audits may not be available, data may exist on certain topics. For example, a GP may have been interested in blood pressure checks at his practice. He may be worried that patients at high risk of developing cardiovascular disease are not having regular blood pressure checks. Whilst he has not defined any standards or formally collected any data, he may have collected a limited amount of pilot data on the last few patients he saw in clinic. As important as such data is, the enthusiasm of someone in the field to help the lead auditor is invaluable to producing a high-quality audit.

Audits of interest

The undertaking of a high-quality audit with robust data collection and important findings will take some effort and it is important that the audit is chosen within a field of interest, not merely because the opportunity presents itself. For example, a FY1 trainee may be interested in a career in surgery but during her intensive care rotation her consultant may suggest an audit looking into tight glycaemic control in patients with sepsis.

Rather than immediately agree to do this, a hybrid option would be to conduct the audit only in patients who have sepsis postoperatively. This would make the audit easier to carry out and also ensure that the findings will be relevant to her aspirations of a future career in surgery. A more difficult scenario would be if she were asked about an audit in a completely unrelated specialty such as psychiatry. It would be up to her to see whether she could justify spending her time on an audit that would be less helpful for her career. It may be wiser to take a step back, e.g. work on the audit but not as the lead auditor, and spend her time more wisely, e.g. trying to get a surgical poster presented at a conference.

Novel ideas

If you are going to initiate an audit within your area of work, it is important to make it novel. There is little use in repeating an audit that has been done many times before unless it is one that is very easy to do (e.g. continuing a previous simple audit to close the loop) or is in an important area, e.g. a national priority. If this is not the case, then it is important that you find an audit that is different enough to attract the eye of future shortlisting and interview panel members.

It may be that you can use your own personal experience and expertise in an otherwise old area, e.g. a doctor who is technologically minded may be interested in the impact of web-based learning or electronic case records in their department. A trainee who is interested in patient attitudes may devise a novel survey to look into attitudes within a field where it is less commonly sought, e.g. should all inpatients on the wards have a consultation from the microbiology team rather than have them simply write their recommendations in the notes?

Multidisciplinary audits

A good audit is one that takes into account a range of ideas and interests related to one issue. An audit can still do this and be very specialised, e.g. evaluating the use of novel blood tests to diagnose malaria may need to take into account the clinicians, microbiology and immunology departments, and a research team within the hospital. A clinical audit can also do this by taking into account the multidisciplinary team, e.g. an audit evaluating the percentage of patients who receive a walking aid after emergency hip replacement could involve an orthopaedic surgeon as the lead auditor, a junior surgeon to collect the data and an occupational therapist to help set the standard and suggest useful interventions.

In addition it may be useful to involve other teams who share a similar problem. For example an audit evaluating patient waiting times in an endocrinology clinic could be expanded to cover respiratory and cardiology patients who all share the same clinic space and receptionist staff. This would make it a more powerful audit and the results could later be broken down to produce data specific to each specialty.

Hot topics

The initiation of a new audit should be in an area of interest and also be novel. A final factor in the choice of topic should be that it is current and cutting edge. This will make it more interesting to potential interview panels. Such topics are straightforward to find and can be done so by simply talking to senior colleagues in the field and searching for recent research articles and reviews.

An alternate method would be to look into relevant specialist organisations for the field of interest. These societies may display information on audit ideas that can be adjusted from a national audit to a small-scale audit within your setting. There may be information of research priorities, recently awarded grants and areas of future interest. As well as specific institutions, national audit societies and other government bodies will have areas of interest that can be applied to an audit.

Publications and presentations

All audits should be carried out with a view to publication. This makes them far more attractive to a short-listing committee. A novel, important or exciting audit will make this easier. The publication may be in the form of a poster at a local conference or an abstract in a related journal.

The audit findings should also be presented to as large a body as possible. This may be the entire GP practice or hospital department but it is important to invite others who may be interested, e.g. managers, members from the local PCT or clinicians from other departments. If there are any formal meetings then the audit should be presented at these, e.g. a regular audit meeting in the hospital or a formal meeting of GP practices within a catchment area. Presentation to such a meeting should be included as part of the description of the audit.

Detailing the audit on a CV or application form

It is important to briefly describe the audit in as succinct terms as possible. A certain level of detail will be helpful as a point of discussion in an interview. For example, do not simply state that you 'carried out an audit into bronchoscopy times in my local hospital and found that the times taken to get a biopsy result were longer in the cases of bronchoscopies than CT-guided biopsies.' Instead, if space on the application form allows it, the audit should be described as follows:

Audit of time taken to get histological diagnosis from lung cancer patients (*150 words*)

I was concerned about the time it took for some patients to get their diagnosis when I worked at St Michael's Hospital as an FY2 trainee in chest medicine. Together with my consultant, I created a standard of 5 days from biopsy to diagnosis, which was based on national guidance from the British Heart and Lung Society. I examined the case notes of 40 patients over a 6-month period and found that although the CT-guided biopsies were generally achieving the standard, only 70% of bronchoscopy biopsies achieved this.

I identified the route of transport as a rate-limiting factor and suggested a standardised method of sample collection and processing. I presented my findings to the monthly lung cancer meeting in the region, which encompassed clinicians and nurses from five local hospitals, and my consultant agreed with my idea for intervention. This has taken place and there will be a re-audit later this year to see if the standard has been achieved.

Sources of further information

Department of Health Clinical Governance: http://www.dh.gov.uk/en/Publichealth/Patientsafety/Clinicalgovernance/index.htm

National Audit Office: http://www.nao.org.uk

Publications

Key aims of this chapter

- Describe in detail the different types of medical publications
- Discuss tips on how to get published as a junior doctor
- Examine non-traditional methods of achieving a publication.

Introduction

Having a published piece to your name is by no means a pre-requisite for getting a job on a specialist training scheme. Most clinicians leaving their foundation years will not have published any medical literature and of those who have, only a small number will have written an article in a respected peer-reviewed journal. However, publications stand out on an application form above many other things. They also show that a candidate has taken the time to pursue something that is challenging and has almost definitely worked towards it in their own time. A publication may serve as a basis for shortlisting applicants or even as an interview question. It may be helpful in guiding the process toward conversations with a topic that may be more familiar to you than the interviewers.

Getting your name published as a medical author can be more straightforward than expected. However, getting a good publication that stands out from the crowd is more challenging and requires thought, hard work and will often need a little thinking outside of the box.

Basics of journal publication

Impact factors

The number of medical journals available to clinicians and researchers in the UK is large and increases every month as new journals are published for the first time. Some journals are universally agreed to be of high quality such as *The Lancet* and *The New England Journal of Medicine*. However, for the vast majority of journals it can be difficult to assess their comparative importance, especially when they have similar titles, e.g. the *Journal of Allergy & Clinical Immunology* and *Clinical Reviews in Allergy & Immunology*. Another example is when looking at region-specific titles, e.g. is it more prestigious to publish your case study in the *South African Medical Journal* or the *Medical Journal of Australia*?

The impact factor is one of a few universally agreed measures of assessing the importance of a scientific or clinical journal. It is a calculation based on the frequency that papers within the journal are cited in other journals over a 2-year period. The rationale for this is that if a journal contains papers that are commonly cited it is likely to be important. Letters to the editor and editorials are not included in this ranking.

---

a = the total number of instances that articles published in 2008 and 2009 were cited by indexed journals during 2010

b = the total number of articles published in 2008 and 2009 in that journal 2010 impact factor = a/b

---

Box 10.1 Calculating an impact factor

In essence, if a journal has an impact factor of 10, it means that on average each article within it was cited 10 times by articles in other publications. Medical journals with high-impact factors (as of 2008) include *The New England Journal of Medicine* (51), *Nature* (31) and *The Lancet* (28). New journals receive their impact factors 2 years after the first publication.

There is some criticism of the rigorous use of impact factors in publishing. Journals can bias the impact factor depending on the type of article they produce, e.g. a review of pulmonary emboli in a clinical journal may be more widely cited than a purely scientific article analysing the proteins involved in forming blood clots in the lungs. However, this does not necessarily mean that the clinical review is superior to the scientific paper.

It may also be that a single highly cited article on pulmonary emboli is alone responsible for raising the impact factor of that journal, which does not necessarily mean that the journal as a whole has improved. However, despite a few alternative methods of ranking, the impact factor is still the most widely used in medicine and senior clinicians and scientists use it regularly to rank their own publication output as well as that of their colleagues.

Authorship criteria

When deciding to write an article for publication it is important to lay out the authorship criteria and positions of names right at the beginning. This will prevent problems between contributors when the article is accepted for publication. In general, authors should be restricted to those who have actually contributed towards the collection of data, analysis of results or writing of the paper. Colleagues who have a smaller role, e.g. bleeding patients for a study or reviewing the final manuscript before publication are usually thanked at the end of the article and not necessarily made authors themselves.

This is not always the case and there are several instances when the rules are bent. It may be that a senior and respected clinician is attached to the department. They may not have done any of the actual work but their name as an author may help improve the chances of acceptance by a journal, particularly if they have written for that journal before. It may also be as a favour to a colleague that it is agreed that they are given authorship. Whilst such practices should not take place, they often do.

The first-named author of any paper should be the person who has contributed the most whilst the last author is typically the most senior member of the group. For example, an ST1 trainee in cardiology may have produced an audit about the use of thrombolysis for myocardial infarcts in their hospital and found that the door-to-needle time in their hospital was far faster than the average for her region. She may want to write this up as a brief paper for a clinical journal and in doing so she would be the first author. Middle authors would include the thrombolysis nurse who helped collect the data, the FY1 doctor on the team who helped write the paper and the ST1 in respiratory medicine who helped analyse the data. The cardiology consultant who initiated the audit and then reviewed the final paper should the last author.

When writing a review with only two authors the accepted positioning of names becomes a little more hazy. In general, the first author will still be the junior doctor who has written the bulk of the article whilst the second author will be the experienced senior clinician who has reviewed the piece and made some changes before submission. However, some senior doctors assume that they should take the first author position and may try and push for it. In all cases where a junior doctor has done the bulk of the work, they should always be positioned as first author. It is important to politely but firmly explain this to any senior doctor who may try and jostle for that position.

Peer review

High-quality journals that accept clinical and scientific papers will have a system of peer review. Two or three experts in the field will be asked to read all submissions to give their opinion on the suitability. They may reject the paper entirely, allow its acceptance with minor changes or they may ask for substantial changes before they will review it again. The reviewers are usually anonymous and independent from each other and will only have the chance to see other comments after the journal has received all reviews. The person submitting the article may have a chance to respond to these comments before the journal editor makes a final decision.

With case studies, abstracts and more concise pieces of work there may be no formal process of peer review but the journal will always have an in-house process to formally score all submissions before making a decision on acceptance. The timescale from submission to decision can be lengthy. If a piece is deemed unsuitable it may be rejected within a matter of days but a lengthy review process can take several weeks or even months.

Editorial style

All journals have their own unique style in terms of article layout, length, reference style and terminology. It is important when submitting for publication that the journal's style is followed closely. For example an FY2 trainee may have seen a case on an interesting patient with Osler–Weber–Rendu syndrome. The case may be very unusual and his consultant may have asked him to write it up as a case study. The first journal that they approach may request that the case study is no more than 1000 words long, has up to ten references and three images.

After writing the case up and submitting it as a case study the journal may review it and reject it, saying that it is not interesting enough. The FY2 trainee may decide to send it to an alternative journal but in this case the style policy is that they want a maximum of 600 words, five references and only one image. It is important that the case study be cut down before it is submitted again otherwise it is likely to be rejected immediately, even before the appropriate subeditor has read it.

Open-access publishing

Whilst the abstract of an article is usually free to view, many journals require subscriptions in order to read the piece in its entirety. This may be in the form of a single one-time payment to one particular article, a time pass to access the entire journal (e.g. 24 hours to review all content) or even a subscription to the journal itself. Most hospital and university libraries have paid subscriptions allowing junior doctors to access the articles from work but there may be restrictions on emailing and printing them off.

Once the article has been written, it should be sent around for informal review prior to submission. This is usually to colleagues familiar with the specialty or type of publication and who will hopefully give a frank assessment of the piece. One this is done, the correct journal for submission should be chosen. This depends on the type of article, the field of interest and the relative importance of the work. *Nature* will not accept a clinical case study of an unusual patient with pulmonary beryllium disease and at the same time *Hospital Doctor* will immediately reject a scientific paper investigating T-cell responses to auto-antigens in the same disease.

Submissions for large journals are almost always carried out online. As well as the article itself, the journal may require any figures, references and conflict of interest statements. There will then be a review process that may take only a few days for some journals but for large complicated scientific papers this process may take several weeks. If a sufficient length of time has passed and there has been no response then an email enquiry may push them along.

If the article is rejected then it is important to ask for feedback to improve the chance of publication elsewhere. It may be that the feedback is unjustified, in which case an appeal letter with a detailed explanation may help change the journal's mind or they may ask another expert reviewer for a further opinion. If the article is accepted pending changes then these should be made as quickly as possible and be resubmitted for publication.

Box 10.2 The publishing process

In other cases the article may need to be paid for but may become free after a period of time.

Open-access journals are a recent type of publication. They aim to allow free reading of all their articles. Research bodies such as the Wellcome Trust and Medical Research Council may insist that their grant holders only publish the products of their research in such journals. The payment costs for publishing the article may be met by advertising, subscription fees or the journal may instead charge the authors to publish their work. The argument for this is that it allows everyone to access research publications whilst opponents of the idea claim that there is not enough money involved to allow the peer review and editorial process that is needed for high-quality cutting-edge publications. Recent examples of open-access journals include those from the Public Library of Science such as *PLOS Medicine* or *PLOS One*.

Types of journal

Basic science journals

Scientists and clinical researchers may choose to publish their work in basic science journals. These can be general, e.g. *Cell* and *Science* or specific to the field of research, e.g. *Journal of Immunology* or *Nature Genetics*. Some of these journals are at the very the top in their field and will have a stringent peer-review process and strict editorial policy. The articles published in these papers are often of basic science and may be the culmination of months or even years of work by a team of clinicians and scientists. In other cases the articles may be editorials that have been specifically commissioned by the journal or short review articles to accompany scientific papers, e.g. the publishing of a new immunology-based method of diagnosing malaria may be accompanied by a review of all recent methods of diagnosis by an expert in the field.

Articles published in these journals may also represent translational work. This is the idea of translating basic science from the laboratory into the clinical setting and vice-versa, e.g. a new genetic-based test to screen for familial bowel cancer may have been developed in the laboratory and this would form the body of the paper. The test may also have been taken into the clinic, where it was used on a family at high risk and this would be mentioned at the end of the article. A number of scientific publications value such research as showing a real-world output of basic science and there are a number of newer journals dedicated to this type of publication, e.g. *Science Translational Medicine*.

Clinical journals

Clinical journals are where the bulk of medical research is published. They can be general, e.g. *The New England Journal of Medicine* and *Annals of Internal Medicine* or more specific, e.g. *Academic Radiology* or *Plastic and Reconstructive Surgery*. These journals are long established and usually have straightforward policies of article submission that need to be adhered to. Some such as *The Lancet* may be published weekly to a high readership and contain articles of high impact whereas other may be less frequent and have lower impact articles, e.g. the pathology journal *Pathologica*, which is published every 2 months.

Clinical studies form the bulk of the articles published in these journals. They may have a basic science element but will generally have a patient-centred slant, e.g. the evaluation of a new type of hip surgery in a large population. There may be clinical trials of new therapies as well as comparison studies between two similar systems, e.g. the efficacy of warfarin versus a new type of anticoagulant in preventing strokes in patients with atrial fibrillation.

Large reviews and case series may also be published in clinical journals. The reviews are often invited rather than simply submitted and the case series may encompass a large number of patients or involve a rare disease. Editorials and opinion pieces are also found in clinical journals and again may be in house or have been specifically commissioned to accompany scientific papers in the same issue.

Medicine-in-practice journals

These journals cover a wide spectrum of medicine. They may be aligned more scientifically, e.g. *The British Medical Journal* or be focused more on the process of practising medicine, e.g. *Hospital Doctor*. They may contain scientific papers but are more likely to cover articles of interest for practising clinicians such as clinical reviews, educational pieces and career information. In addition, they may contain political pieces, editorials and news items. Some of this is not peer-reviewed publishing but will still have to make it through the editorial policy of the journal.

These journals are still usually in paper format but may have a large presence on the Internet with added information, extra articles that have not made it into the paper edition and links to other resources. Some of these publications require a paid subscription whilst others rely purely on advertising for revenue and are distributed freely.

Lifestyle journals

These journals are primarily focused on the lives of doctors rather than their work. They are unlikely to contain scientific articles and are more focused on career advice, politics, editorials, reviews and lifestyle pieces. Examples include *Junior Doctor* and *GP* magazine. These journals tend to be freely distributed and rely on advertising and commercial tie-ins to create revenue. The level of peer review is lower here but in contrast to some of the other journals they may not accept submissions on a regular basis but use in-house staff to produce much of their work.

How to get published

There are a number of ways in which to get your article published in a medical journal whilst still a junior doctor. Some of these involve hard work whilst others involve serendipity, merely being there at the right place at the right time. There are a myriad of opportunities to publish work and it is often a case of actively seeking out those possibilities.

Research from medical school

A number of junior doctors will have undertaken a research project during medical school, e.g. as part of an intercalated degree. This may have resulted in a publication, but if not it is important to ensure that any scientific work has not been wasted. There may be project data that has been completed but that has not been published. This is usually due to lack of time in medical school or lack of initiative on the part of the student or the research team. If unsure, the original group leader should be contacted and a meeting set up to go over any data with a specific view to publication of any results.

Often, the work may have been brief but may have continued with other students or scientists after the initial data has been gathered. One way of finding this out would be to again approach the group and ask if the work has been taken forward. Any future publication that results from work undertaken by a project student should ideally list them as an author of the paper, though not necessarily as the first author.

It may be that no data of relevance was produced during medical school but there are still opportunities for publication, e.g. a FY1 trainee may have undertaken a project looking for cellular responses to atypical mycobacteria. Although the project took 3 months and produced some data, the output was not robust and no one has taken that work forward. However, during that time she adapted slightly the standard method of counting cells with a microscope to make it faster for her to do. She discusses this with her BSc supervisor and they agree to write a short article and submit it to a low-impact factor journal, explaining her faster method. This gets published and although it will not be groundbreaking research, it shows that she had the initiative to do something differently and take this forward to write it up.

Case studies

These are a popular way of publishing as a junior doctor. These can involve a single rare condition, the unusual presentation of a common condition or a series of conditions. It is important to keep an eye out for such cases as it may be that they present to other teams, e.g. ST trainees in medicine sitting the final part of their membership exams are a good source of knowledge of unusual cases and can be relied upon to provide their details. Although the time on the wards in any given specialty as a junior doctor is limited, it is important to note that senior doctors within the team may have specific patients that they have always wanted to write up. These may be patients that they have seen in clinic on a regular basis or those who were admitted with an unusual diagnosis. It is important to ask your consultant or GP trainers if they have any such patients in mind.

Once a case has been found, it is vital to find an angle that makes it special and hence publishable. Even rare diseases can be found in textbooks so they have to be different, e.g. a GP trainee asks a partner in the practice if she has any interesting patients whom he would like to write up. She tells him that they have seen two patients in the last few years with Addison's disease that were both initially missed as they presented with an unusual skin complaint as their main problem. The trainee then has to read thoroughly the notes to see if they are indeed interesting and then carry out a literature search to look for similar cases. Once he is convinced that they do warrant writing up he should do so and ask the partner for her advice and review before they submit it together.

Prior to submission, consent should be granted from all patients involved. Although the patient will only ever be referred to by their initials, it is still important to gain this consent, particularly if images or other investigations are being shown. The case study should then be submitted to an appropriate journal and research needs to be carried out to see which is suitable. Some journals prefer shorter pieces whereas others look for formal studies with detailed investigations and this should be taken into account when drafting the article.

A number of new on-line journals have recently sprung up to deal solely with case reports, e.g. *BMJ Case Reports*. Whilst there is increased opportunity for publishing in these journals, the fee associated with such submissions may make them less attractive on a shortlisting form.

Educational pieces

These are pieces that may have started off as case studies but were found to have insufficient material to warrant a publication. Often they will simply be a picture such as an unusual CT-scan or ECG. It is important to target these appropriately, e.g. a medical student journal may be interested in a chest x-ray showing dextrocardia but this would not be able to find its way into a journal for practising clinicians. Some journals actively request such pieces and the submissions should be targeted towards those. Other journals have themed issues and may welcome a relevant short piece as a filler in between lengthier papers.

Scientific research

Many hospitals and GPs in urban areas are associated with teaching hospitals and universities. Senior clinicians here often have honorary contracts with academic institutions and are actively involved with recruiting for studies and carrying out experimental work, and there is often ample opportunity to get involved.

Lecturers and Clinical Fellows are clinicians who also undertake research. In the case of an ST trainee studying for a PhD this may be full-time research but in the case of an honorary consultant this may be part time. They are often very keen to persuade more junior doctors to enter research and as a result will often be helpful in forming collaborations. For example, an Oncology Fellow may need to take blood samples from a specific number of patients with a particular cancer but finds it difficult to prioritise patient samples with their laboratory work. An FY2 trainee may spend an entire year in that hospital and could contact the Fellow whenever they see a particular case that fits the study criteria. This help should result in at least a mention of thanks on any resulting publications but if the collaboration extends further, e.g. stratifying the demographic data of the patients then it may result in an authorship.

Researchers should also be sought out through contacts within the hospital or general practice. This will take some initiative but may be fruitful, e.g. an ST2 in a busy inner city hospital may be interested in the large caseload of tuberculosis patients at the chest clinic. There may not be ongoing research but by contacting an affiliated university research department she may find a TB research team that needs to recruit blood and bronchoscopy samples for their ongoing research. A collaboration could be formed whereby samples from her outpatient clinic are sent to the University. She could then be entitled to authorship on any publications resulting from the use of those clinical samples.

Clinical research

The majority of research published by junior doctors falls into this category. Spending time on the wards and in general practice allows doctors to get ideas for a number of different types of clinical article. Senior doctors are usually keen to publish clinical research in their field and often have ideas for studies that they wish to pursue, e.g. a general surgeon may specialise in laproscopic surgery and he may have been to a conference advocating a new type of instrument for cholecystectomy. One idea to investigate this would be to compare the standard and new types of equipment in a randomised trial. After getting the appropriate ethical approval he may decide that he only needs to perform five operations in each arm of the study. Whilst he would perform the operations himself, he may ask his FY2 trainee to do the background research and draft the paper.

It may be that a junior doctor notices that a particular system in his department is different to the usual practice and decides to write about this, e.g. an FY2 trainee in paediatrics may note that all parents of children in the outpatient allergy clinic are sent allergy leaflets by post along with the appointment letter, which gives them a chance to read it before seeing the doctor. He may wonder if this is helpful and decides to give out a questionnaire to parents as they arrive in clinic. The questionnaire, leaflets and thoughts behind the process could be written up as a clinical opinion piece with his consultant and used to advocate the benefits of patient information for parents of allergy sufferers.

Another common form of collaborative clinical publishing is to write a review of the literature, e.g. a respiratory physician may be interested in pulmonary emboli and may wish to write a review of the different treatment modalities with the assistance of her ST1 trainee. Whilst she may write a very rough sketch the ST1 will be asked to write the first draft of the review and bring it back for further work. Clinical reviews are usually discussed prior to submission and all ideas for up-to-date articles should be pitched to the appropriate journal.

Audits

An audit of high enough quality can act as a potential submission for publication. As well as being well written it should evaluate a novel or important issue. To increase the chances of acceptance for publication it should incorporate interventions that are proven to increase the outcome after re-evaluation of the audit. It could then be submitted as a short article or incorporated into related research and form part of a larger paper. It is worth noting which journals publish audit and what the editorial policy for these publications is. Some journals such as *Clinical Audit* are dedicated purely to audit but acceptance here may be associated with large publishing fees, especially if the journal is an open-source type.

Opinion pieces and personal viewpoints

These are often published on a regular basis as fillers in between other articles. Most clinical journals, including high-impact publications such as *The New England Journal of Medicine*, publish such pieces in every issue. They can often be submitted unsolicited and may be accepted but only published when a piece is needed, which may be several months after acceptance.

In order to increase the chances of publication, it may be helpful to target such a piece to a journal with a themed issue, e.g. the *Journal of the American Medical Association* may announce that they are looking for research on doctors' working hours and how it affects their lifestyle. An FY2 trainee may wish to write a piece comparing the hours of a junior doctor in the UK with that of her colleagues in the USA and use her personal experiences as a starting point. When writing about particular patients it is vital to be as confidential as possible; use initials only and minimise the personal non-medical details that could be used to identify them.

Editorials and letters to the editor

It is unlikely that a junior doctor would be invited to write an editorial in a peer-reviewed journal unless the publication was specifically looking for their viewpoint, e.g. in the case of a political editorial discussing the working time directive or on-call duties in relation to hospital at night. Another reason for an invitation would be if they had a special type of experience, e.g. a strong research background in a particular area.

Letters to the editor, however, are often written by junior doctors, many in response to a particular article and may give an alternative view, e.g. an ST2 trainee in ophthalmology reads about a review article discussing a new type of cataract surgery. She feels that the article has missed out a key side effect that she has seen in her practice. She discusses this with her consultant and they agree to write a brief letter in response, stating that whilst the review was very good, it failed to mention something that they had seen in their own clinical practice.

Poster presentations

Although these are not publications in the strictest sense they are a method for presenting work to a national or international forum. They are often presented in the form of an abstract and detail research of a basic science or clinical nature, but can also convey audit results and even personal viewpoints. They can be detailed on the CV in much the same way as a written publication and so authorship rules are similar. Conferences that ask for poster submissions usually have a high rate of acceptance as it means that the organisers are guaranteed to get both the content for their poster sessions and conference fees paid for by the people attending to present their poster.

Scholarships and travel awards from the appropriate medical societies are often available but this depends on the type and prestige of the conference, e.g. the *British Lung Foundation* may have scholarships to support poster presentations at the *American Thoracic Society* annual meeting but not to the British or European equivalents.

Book chapters

An alternative to publication in a peer-reviewed journal is to write a chapter for a medical book. Junior doctors can write chapters for a number of different types of books including those aimed at junior doctors or at medical students, e.g. lifestyle books or revision texts. For textbooks senior authors are required but they may have junior co-authors who are asked to write the first draft of the chapter.

Publishing houses may have details of upcoming books where the editors are still looking for chapter authors. An other method is to contact Clinical

Research Fellows at academic institutions, who will invariably know of books that are in the process of being written where editors are searching for junior co-authors.

Publishing in your field

As with audit, it is important to try to publish in a field that will have long-term career implications. Whilst all authorships are important the position can be less important than the topic, e.g. an FY2 trainee wishing to specialise in oncology may benefit more from being a middle author on a clinical paper investigating anti-emetic therapies for patients undergoing aggressive chemotherapy than if he were the first author on a review of cognitive behavioural therapy. When time is limited it is more important to pursue avenues of relevance.

Persuading editors to publish your piece

The article must be important, timely and of clinical or scientific relevance. For example, a clinical review on heart disease may be welcomed if the Government has recently announced large increases in the research budget for this type of illness. On the other hand, a review of pneumonia that is submitted to a journal that has recently published several similar pieces may be rejected even if it is better written than previous work.

Once ready for submission, the article must match the desired style for that section of the journal. Assuming that the piece is of scientific or clinical interest, editors who find that a submission is too long, is poorly written or does not match the required template may reject the piece outright rather than spend time detailing the required changes.

If allowed, a cover letter should be always submitted along with the article. This should be concise but nevertheless explain in exact detail why the research is cutting edge, why it has advantages over recent competitors and why it should be published in this particular journal. For example, a review of acute leukaemia may explain that not only have there been no recent reviews of high standard but that the last one of note was published in the same journal more than 10 years ago and that there have been many changes in the intervening time. A personal piece could be supported by a letter stating that it is in line with other specific pieces published in the same journal and that it would be suitable for a particular upcoming themed issue.

If the piece is rejected outright it is important to get feedback. This may help you make the case for publication to the same journal (if the reviewers' feedback is strongly disagreed with) or it may help change the article before submission elsewhere. Unless expressly asked in the submission process it should not be mentioned that the article has been previously sent to a different publication. Journal editors do not like being anybody's second choice.

Alternative forms of publication

Medical journalism

Becoming involved with medical journalism is an alternative form of getting published. A number of journals actively seek full- or part-time journalists, e.g. the *British Medical Journal* has traditionally employed one *Clegg Scholar* each year. This is often a doctor-in-training who leaves clinical practice for a period to write for them full time. Journals such as *Junior Doctor* magazine welcome part-time writers as well as submission of non-scientific pieces such as editorials, news articles and opinion pieces. The editor of such journals should always be contacted prior to submission as they may want to see evidence of a standard of journalism or the draft version of a piece before they agree to commission an article.

Editorials and editorial boards

In addition to writing articles it is sometimes possible to sit on the editorial boards of journals. These may be journals that are dedicated to more junior trainees such as *Junior Doctor* or the *Student BMJ* or they may be clinical journals that are actively seeking junior editorial members. These positions are usually widely advertised. Participating on such boards may require physical attendance at regular meetings but they are increasingly taking place in a virtual environment, e.g. members are emailed pieces and can then upload their opinions and views to a central server. Editorial board members have their names published in the print versions of the journal and the position is extremely desirable on a CV.

Online publishing

A number of traditional journals have websites that publish articles that may not have been of high enough standard to make the print version but nonetheless warrant publication. These can be presented on a CV in a similar way to a paper publication but sometimes have an 'e' in front of the journal title to indicate that they have been published electronically.

In addition to traditional journals, some publications are purely web based and these may have a higher rate of acceptance but these are often limited to the more technical specialties, e.g. *Internet Journal of Anesthesiology*. Sites such as *emedicine* and *uptodate* also publish clinical material on the web and actively seek out both senior and junior authors.

Detailing the publication on a CV or application form

If allowed, it is important to concisely detail the publication. At a senior level a clinician may have a number of publications and it may simply be a case of listing them with the important ones highlighted. For a junior doctor who might have just one publication it is useful to detail the level of their involvement in the article. This will be useful to a short-listing panel who may see a number of similar CVs:

> *Stroke in London: A review of the existing proformas.* **Jameson A**, *Mehta C and Collins S. Journal of Stroke rehabilitation. 2009 Nov 10;516(7):929–938.*

> *I was the first author for this article, which was published in a peer-reviewed journal last year. I examined a number of different stroke proformas from hospitals across London. Once I had collected the data, I analysed the results and created a template for a hypothetical stroke proforma that encompassed a number of different issues. I wrote the first draft of the paper, which was then reviewed by the last author (Professor S. Collins) prior to submission.*

Sources of further information

Platform for journal rankings: http://isiwebofknowledge.com/sciencegateway.org/rank/index.html

Directory of open access journals: http://www.doaj.org/uib.no/isf/guide/journal.htm

List of medical journals from the US national Library of Medicine and National Institutes of Health: http://www.ncbi.nlm.nih.gov/journals

Index

duties of a doctor 33, 34
effective communication
117
management of adverse
events 111
person specification,
foundation
programme 32
preparation for GP
training assessment
123, 128
team working 37–8

H

haematology, pros/cons of
working in 11
health promotion, training in
foundation years 43
HIV medicine, pros/cons of
working in 11
hospital consultants
attitude to colleague,
specialty training
application 94–5
remuneration 3, 4
teaching responsibilities
4
workload 3

I

immunology, pros/cons of
working in 12
impact factors, journals
164–5, 169
calculation 164
income see remuneration
induction, foundation
programmes 43
infectious diseases, pros/
cons of working in 11
initiative, using
publishing research from
medical school 171
in specialty training
application form 91–2
insurance companies 7
intensive care medicine,
pros/cons of working
in 12
intercalated degrees 16, 31,
86, 109, 110, 170
inter-deanery transfers 6,
56–7, 72
interests (other), specialty
training application
form 89–90

interpersonal skills,
specialty training
application form
90–1
interviews (job) xi
specialty training see
specialty training
interviews
investigation, audit vs 147

J

job satisfaction 2
job vacancies 67
advertising see
advertising of
vacancies/posts
journal(s)
acceptance for publication
165
authorship criteria
165–6
basic facts/principles
164–8
basic science 168–9
clinical 169
cover letter 176
editorial(s) 168, 174–5,
177
editorial boards 177
editorial style 166–7, 176
impact factors 164–5, 169
informal review before
submission 167
letters to editor 174–5
lifestyle 170
medicine-in-practice
169–70
online 172, 177–8
online submission 167
open-access 167–8
peer review 166
persuading editors to
publish 176–7
rejection of article/paper
166, 167, 176–7
translation work (from
laboratory to clinic)
168–9
types 168–70
journalism, medical 4, 5,
177

K

knowledge-based
assessments (exit
exams) 132

L

The Lancet 164, 169
lead auditor 148, 153, 156,
159
'lead' deanery 66
learning, life-long see
continual learning
learning needs, personal
development plan
51–2
leave, for study 138
FY1 and FY2 55
legal issues, training in
foundation years 43
life-long learning see
continual learning
lifestyle journals 170
literature review 173–4
litigation 7
location
foundation programmes
26, 27
selection assessment
centre 124
specialty training posts
68–9
long-term strategy/career
path xi
postgraduate exam timing
135
publishing in own field
176
in specialty training
application form 89

M

management, questions
at specialty training
interview 112
Masters degrees 110, 132
MBPhD 110
medical insurance 4
medical journalism 4, 5, 177
medical schools, impact
on foundation
programme
applications 26
medicine, postgraduate
exam format 139–40
medicine-in-practice journals
169–70
meetings/conferences
leave for attending 138
presentations, questions
about 79–80
memory lapse 114

microbiology, pros/cons of working in 12
mini-clinical evaluation exercise (mini-CEX) 45, 48, 49
mini-PAT (peer assessment tool) 45, 47–8
minor surgery, courses on 54
Modernising Medical Careers (MMC) xi, 5, 43, 59, 132
'morbidity and mortality' meetings, audit 152
MRCP exam 131
multidisciplinary fields, audits in 149
MultiDisciplinary Meeting (MDT) 48
multiple choice questions (MCQs) 133–4
    best of five format 133
    databases 136–7
    practice for 133–4
    specialty-specific exams 139, 140, 141, 143
multiple matching test 122–4
    see also general practitioners (GPs) recruitment
multi-source feedback (MSF) 45, 47–8

N
National Office for GP Recruitment 75, 128
National Person Specification, GP recruitment 122, 128
Nature 164
negative marking 123, 133
neurology, pros/cons of working in 12
neurosurgery, pros/cons of working in 13
The New England Journal of Medicine 164, 169, 174
NHS Executive, clinical audit definition 146
NHS Jobs 67
NICE, clinical audit definition 146

non-academic achievements, in foundation programme application 39
non-consultant posts 7
non-UK doctors
    PLAB exam 133
    specialty training 72

O
objective structured clinical examination (OSCE) 54, 134–5
    specialty-specific exams 140, 143
obstetrics and gynaecology
    postgraduate exam format 143
    pros/cons of working in 13
on-call
    private practice and 7
    workload and working hours 3
oncology, pros/cons of working in 12
online courses, postgraduate exam revision 136–7
online publishing 172, 177–8
open-access publishing 167–8
ophthalmology, pros/cons of working in 13
opinion pieces, publication 174
oral and maxillofacial surgery, pros/cons of working in 13
organisational skills, in specialty training application form 81–2
orthopaedics 59
    pros/cons of working in 14
out-of-programme (OOP) experiences 72
overseas doctors
    PLAB exam 133
    specialty training 72
overseas exams/ qualifications 132–3
overseas students, foundation programmes 28
overseas training 57

P
PACES (MRCP Part 2 Clinical Examination) 139–40
paediatrics 54
    postgraduate exam format 141
palliative care, pros/cons of working in 14
part-time medicine 5–6
pathology
    postgraduate exam format 143–4
    pros/cons of working in 12
patient care, audit issue selection 154
patient-centred audit 152–3
patient needs, question in foundation programme application 33–5
patient safety, training in foundation years 42
pay see remuneration
pay awards 3–4
peer review 166
personal attributes, in foundation programme application 30, 34
personal development plan 51–2
personalised revision notes 137
person specifications
    for core medical training 64–5
    for foundation programme application 29–31, 32, 38
    for GP training 122, 126, 128
    personal development plan and 52
    for specialty training 63–5, 75
    difficult questions 115–16
    testing, at interviews 114, 115
PhD 17, 72, 109, 172
PLAB (Professional and Linguistic Assessments Board) 133